AF594902

THE CURE AT WALDEN POND

THE CURE AT WALDEN POND

A Guide to Recovering Our Humanity

THOMAS MOORE

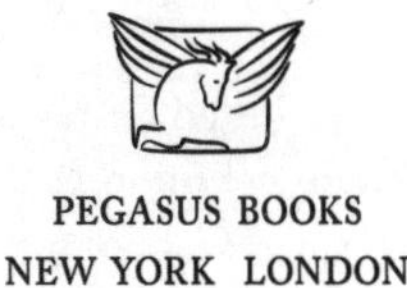

PEGASUS BOOKS
NEW YORK LONDON

To my brother, Jim

THE CURE AT WALDEN POND

Pegasus Books, Ltd.
148 West 37th Street, 12th Floor
New York, NY 10018

First Pegasus Books cloth edition July 2026

Interior design by Maria Fernandez

Library of Congress Cataloging-in-Publication Data is available.

ISBN: 979-8-89710-129-0

10 9 8 7 6 5 4 3 2 1

Printed in the United States of America
Distributed by Simon & Schuster
www.pegasusbooks.com

Thoreau was a surprising fellow—he is not easily grasped—he is elusive: yet he is one of the native forces.

—Walt Whitman[1]

Contents

INTRODUCTION

On July 4, 1845, an ardent naturalist and pencil maker left his home in Concord, Massachusetts, to take his life a step forward by conducting an experiment in living next to a small lake, which in New England is called a pond. Walden Pond is just two miles from Concord, and Henry David Thoreau would spend just two years on his experiment. Thoreau was not heroic in this adventure—just the opposite—he wanted to do something simple to root his life in his world. It resulted in one of the most famous American books, *Walden*, and, I believe, could offer us today a blueprint for helping the entire planet come of age and find its maturity.

The point of this book is that we could all deepen our lives, and indeed sanctify them, by following Thoreau's method, but always in our own way. Being individual and eccentric is part of the method. I consider that he and I are both natural theologians, creating a religious life, even a monk's life, in the secular environment. For me, his real strength lies in his ability to look at ordinary things and see myth, the sacred, and the gods.

We, too, can find our equivalent of a Walden Pond and sense some distance from conventional society, asking Thoreau's essential question: At the end of this generation, will we feel that we made the right choices and did we really live meaningful and worthwhile lives? Imitating Thoreau, we could experiment with literal forms of retreat, or we could step back in imagination and wonder how life could be different, and better. I hope this book is a Walden Pond for you.

Thoreau did not live an abstract life. He did not teach a high-minded philosophy. He put together a simple yet philosophical lifestyle as he walked the woods and paddled his boat. The perch in the rivers, the mice in his cabin, and the birds flying overhead contributed to his thinking. He enjoyed a combination of virtues that we could use today: deep acquaintance with the world around him and a background in philosophical and spiritual teachings. This book could take you on a brief retreat and inspire you, just as Thoreau was inspired "to live more deliberately."

This book is not *about* Thoreau; rather, it turns to him and his cabin by the lake for lessons in how to renew our lives. I am not an expert on Thoreau. Here, I am in conversation with him. I hope to show you that Thoreau's vision could help you establish your own philosophy of life. From the beginning I thought of this work as a cure for both of us, me and the reader, as the Walden in the woods cured Thoreau. I would like this book to be a therapy for our world as it suffers global mental health issues that are at the root of our social problems. I envision Thoreau not only as the intense naturalist he was but also as a probing depth psychologist.

Mainly I address this book to the individual person trying to adjust to this rapidly changing world and its dehumanizing trend. Is there a way we can live, not demonizing technology, but giving it a human context and purpose in our lives? Can we educate ourselves, respond to our illnesses, and live in a world less technical and more soulful? Thoreau was an eccentric, to say the least. Can we set ourselves apart from the majority, which buys too readily into the mechanical approaches to modern life? Can we search our wounded hearts and find a cure and live in peace? Can we lovingly detach ourselves from the soulless aspects of modern life and manifest an alternative?

I believe that widespread depression, marital difficulties, and a variety of anxieties are largely due to the cultural climate, its lack of human scale. Most analyses of our situation are too superficial and fail to penetrate to the deep philosophical and spiritual roots of our disarray. There is a cure for us all at Walden Pond, and it has to do with allowing nature to shape our values and to give us an alternative way of living. The way we are doing it now is too much like suicide.

Henry David Thoreau recommended simplicity, for sure, but he was a complicated man. He was educated at Harvard, was good at languages, read broadly, and wrote with a refined style. He could spend half a day in a boat and the rest reading and writing intensely. He could go huckleberrying and then give a lecture. He appreciated wildness but also carved out a life of tranquility. There may be a tendency among some to dismiss Thoreau because of his reputation for roughness, but they could discover his love of language and ideas and even his creative successes in technology, as he ingeniously perfected pencils for his family's business.

My sense of Thoreau's mission does not go in the direction of environmentalism, although you can easily extract that element from his biography and writings. Foremost, he was in search of a way of life that would fulfill his nature, and this is precisely what I think is needed in our world today. We could learn how to support every person on the planet in discovering who they are and how they can shape their lives accordingly. This process is not only fulfilling, but calming. It allows a person to love and appreciate others, whether a life partner or a person speaking a different language on the other side of the world.

We have not yet reached a point in our evolution where we want every person on the planet to be fulfilled and then make that happen. If we felt that way, how could we have wars? We would be dedicated to the apotheosis of every human being, their complete and joyful self-realization. Everyone in their own way on the path of Henry David Thoreau.

We can also learn the subtle lesson from Thoreau that to find yourself you could not do better than to become intimate with the natural world, especially where you live. Thoreau did not go into nature either as a feral misanthrope or as an investigative scientist. He went as someone who wanted to learn from intimacy with the wild and from its mysteries who he was and what he was supposed to do with his life. To follow Thoreau, you keep nature close to town and spend time in it with an open mind. Then you discover, mysteriously, your own nature and know how to live. You learn that the uncanny ways of plants, trees, and animals are your own. By becoming intimate with the natural world, you become intimate with yourself.

Thoreau was so interested in religion and the quest for divinity that I think of him as a theologian. Frequently he said that Walden Pond was the Ganges and that the Rivers of Paradise ran through it. He called himself a yogi. He said that his sacraments included rising early, eating with restraint, and going for a swim. He was not afraid of death because he knew that he was divine. He knew this from observing perch in a stream and noticing the unmanaged dispersal of seeds around the world. He said he was so spiritual that when he died, the undertaker would not have anything to bury.

Thoreau was full of contradictions: A book-loving, idea-hungry naturalist; a music lover who preferred to listen to the hum of telegraph wires than to go to the Boston Symphony; a mountain climber who recommended not getting to the top. He was devoted to the imagination and had a sophisticated psychoanalytic understanding of it. He talked about a mountain that guided him, although it existed only in his imagination. In this, Thoreau was both premodern and postmodern.

Thoreau was ahead of his time and always behind it. He did not belong to his own world, and yet he strongly advocated living in your own time. This, I say, is a model for attaining world peace and for catching up with our own time. It is backward to fight wars and allow children to suffer in them and to maintain a society of extreme wealth against dire poverty. We have not caught up with ourselves, and we are not living the life a twenty-first-century society should have attained by now. It is not worthy of us to try to live in the future when we have not yet attained life in the present.

It is worth reading Thoreau to see how he boated, hiked, climbed, and berry-picked his way to himself and his time. You don't have to become a full-time kayaker, but you could discover your own unique way in the ordinary world in front of you. The idea is not only to learn from nature but also to discover your natural self, your own laws, and your own path to fulfillment. Once there, you can help others do the same and then enjoy a world inspired by Concord.

1

BLUE ANGELS

I have a great deal of company in my house; especially in the morning, when nobody calls. Let me suggest a few comparisons, that some one may convey an idea of my situation. I am no more lonely than the loon in the pond that laughs so loud, or than Walden Pond itself. What company has that lonely lake, I pray? And yet it has not the blue devils, but the blue angels in it, in the azure tint of its waters. . . . I am no more lonely than a single mullein or dandelion in a pasture, or a bean leaf, or sorrel, or a horse fly, or a bumble-bee. I am no more lonely than the Mill Brook, or a weathercock, or the Northstar, or the south wind, or an April shower, or a January thaw, or the first spider in a new house.[1]

—Henry David Thoreau, *Walden*

Henry David Thoreau often writes about his companions in the world of nature. He is not just poetizing, but vividly sensing the world as a family. For him, all those beings he lists are not to be considered objectively and distantly; they are lovers and cousins and neighbors. They relate to each other and to him. How could he be lonely in such a world?

We know more about nature than Thoreau did, and yet we seem to be less intimate with it. We have remarkable tools to work with and a history of expert analysis, yet we would probably hesitate to say with Thoreau, St. Francis of Assisi, and Black Elk, natural mystics, that the animals are our cousins. We are proud of the classical formula in which we are rational animals and find it difficult to be close to animals that do not communicate the way we do.

Thoreau hints that the loneliness of modern life is due not only to estrangement from our fellow humans but also to our failure to feel a natural closeness with the animals, birds, and fish who share our planetary home. They are all around us, but we do not take advantage of their presence by fostering relationships and intimacies. Except, of course, for pets. But our extravagance with pets may indicate how estranged we are from wild animals. We are lonely not only for people, but for the other creatures and even things that populate our world, for wilderness and wildness.

A beloved tree or even a well-crafted tool that you do not want to part with could save you from painful loneliness. Sometimes having an animal nearby or an object that has special meaning can give you a feeling of relationship or intimacy. It will take an effort from you to maintain the connection, while the animal or thing offers itself by being there in its own way.

Thoreau's way of perceiving the world allows him to be free of loneliness by living in a world full of personality. To satisfy his need for intimacy and connection, he requires not only humans but also the whole world of things. Here is a suggestion for all of us who may feel lonely: Maybe we should seek a medicine for our loneliness not only among people, but in nature and amid things that also can have a personality.

Among my tools I have an electric drill that my father gave me when I was in my teens. When I see and hold it now, I have clear memories of him using it expertly and showing me how to handle it. When I grab it now for a task, I remember my father vividly and the drill seems to have a pulse, as though it were alive. Friends wonder why I don't get a new drill, but I can't part with it. Through my father we have a special relationship.

Like Thoreau, we can find relief from any unwanted solitude by initiating a relationship to the things of the world. A relationship of interest and love could replace the current habits of exploitation and consumption. We know how bad it feels to be used by another person, but we don't seem to understand that the world might also feel bad, so to speak, by the loveless way we use and abuse it. Loving the world could give rise to care, and we could care for the things in our homes and towns instead of neglecting their needs. In return, they offer relationship and intimacy.

Take a walk down a city street or a small town and notice how neglected the buildings, roads, and sidewalks are. If we loved them, we might be unsettled by their disrepair. If we could feel some empathy for them, we might feel an intimacy with them and even sense their love coming back.

When I was a child, I would spend summers on a farm in the Finger Lakes region of New York State, in an old farmhouse that had no running water. My uncles cooked on a smelly kerosene stove. Long rifles leaned against an old oak buffet in the kitchen, making you wonder if the Battles of Lexington and Concord had yet to be fought. An ancient out-of-tune piano stood in the haze of a musty parlor. The family loved that house, so that even today, when the house and barn and outbuildings are collapsed and melting into the earth, my cousins and I still visit that sacred spot and reverently pore over the detritus of glorious years gone by.

I have no doubt that the ruins of that farm take considerable joy and immortality from our visit and as others in the family look lovingly at old photos of it and feel warm in the memories of life in that hallowed place. In the small book-lined room in my own house, where I have been writing for several years now, hangs a painting by my Uncle Jack of that farmhouse, and when I look at it, almost daily, as I enter the room, I am reminded of how I loved the place and its objects. That painting, hanging low in a corner now, is like the blue angels shooting over Walden Pond. It sanctifies the room and the large quantity of soul it contains saturates my head and lubricates my hands as I write.

Maybe that painting speaks only to me, the only one left in the family to know that farmhouse, but it puts a glow on my room and into my heart and from there into words appearing on the pages. Loving the objects in our world humanizes us, and isn't that the primary ingredient lacking in modern life? Humanity.

We need not only more advanced tools for our daily lives but also a better and more intimate relationship with them. I still have a clear memory of my Uncle Tom, the farmer, sharpening the blades of the large, wheeled cutter that he employed to mow hay in five-acre fields. The sharpener was a grinding stone with no electrical power and had been used for decades. He powered it with his feet on a treadle. That well-worn stone was like a handyman that Uncle Tom could depend on to keep his farm equipment at their best. That sharpener is now an antique, but there is no reason why today we can't have good relationships with our tools, as my Uncle Tom did, and lovingly care for them.

Thoreau is saying that he is not alone in the world, just as the North Star or a southerly wind are not alone or lonely, because they are a convivial part of the natural community of things. No matter how much space you have around you, no matter how rare it is for people to visit you, you live in a world of friends and relatives, so many that it is absurd to think that you could ever be alone. But you must make friends with this world's inhabitants and get to know them and see their beauty and the intricate role they play in the great web of things. You need to open your heart to them.

Our loneliness does not come from a lack of friends, but from not recognizing the objects in our world as friendly neighbors. We treat these neighbors heartlessly, as though they had no capacity for relationship. We inspect them and improve them endlessly, and then we wonder why so much of our environment is poisonous and trashy. It is angry at our brash, intrusive incursions into its privacy and sensitivities.

We do not have a warm and intimate dialogue with our things; instead, we dissect them and use technology to keep them up to date. Or we neglect them and do not offer them nourishment, like food and drink. Nor do we listen to their complaints or needs. Especially today, when a thing no longer works perfectly, we could repair it. Instead, we put it in the trash.

Not only does Thoreau list the many things of nature that keep him company and tend his potential loneliness, he senses the sacred in a world that most of us consider secular. Looking over the waters of Walden Pond, he spots blue angels in the azure tints of its waves. It would not take much for us to see blue angels in our world, but we would have to enter that level of reality where images are real. Even in a world of science and widespread materialism, angels can be found.

Thoreau's way of being religious is his strongest virtue and perhaps the quality most difficult to appreciate in our modern secular age. His blue angels of Walden represent only one of many references in his work to a nonsectarian, natural, and often informal religious eye. He claims that his world, with all its secularism, is saturated with the divine. In the Sufi tradition, Kabir said, "I laughed when I heard of a fish in the water who was thirsty." Thoreau had no thirst for God, as he knew he was surrounded by the divine.

2

FLUTTERING

We can only live healthily the life the gods assign us. I must receive my life as passively as the willow leaf that flutters over the brook. I must not be for myself, but God's work, and that is always good. I will wait the breezes patiently, and grow as nature shall determine.[1]

—Henry David Thoreau, journal entry, March 11, 1842

Life is a series of invitations and challenges that come to us as faint physical prompts or as signs and signals in the everyday world. The first strong push for me came when I was just thirteen years old. I became infatuated with the Catholic priesthood that I witnessed in the school and church my family attended, and, against my parents' desire, I left home to pursue the dream of becoming a priest.

The impetus then was a burning vision of my future. It had to be powerful because I left behind a big warm family that I loved, only to go off into a world of fantasy. I stayed with that monastic life, which had its pleasures and its harshness as well, for thirteen years, and then I noticed signs that I wasn't cut out for it after all. Abruptly, I left the monastery with no prospects and no money, but with the certainty that I was being led in a different direction.

When I look back now, I see how those years as a monk prepared me for my current life as a writer and teacher. It is as though someone had a plan for me, which all makes sense now in my eighties—each separate, improbable piece of it. I could never have planned this life, and yet it seems perfect, nothing out of place. My job was to stay alert for signs of change and have the willingness to move on when the signals were clear.

We do not make our lives with our own intentions and expectations. We are made, and it is our job to pay attention to the clues we need to get where we want to go. Thoreau says, "I will wait the breezes patiently." We don't live, we are lived. We don't choose our life plan, we are chosen by it. In many medieval paintings, the West Wind, Zephyr, blows in new life. When I feel such a breeze, I say to myself, "The guiding wind is stirring once again. It is time to flutter."

This approach to life contradicts the modern way in which the *I* is supreme. *I* am in charge. *I* invent my life as I go. It might be better to wait for a sign and read the omens carefully. The willingness to be led is the essence of religion, acknowledging another will. "Thy will be done." "Inshallah." A prayer from the Chinook people says it all quite briefly and in the spirit of Thoreau:

> May all I say and all I think
> be in harmony with thee,
> God within me,
> God beyond me,
> maker of the trees.

What is behind it all? The one who made the trees. Say no more. I often meditate on the tall trees that surround my house, considering them in light of the Chinook prayer. Acknowledgment of the other, not defined and not personalized, keeps a person human, because being human requires connection with another will. From this dialogue comes a life that fits snugly with the needs of a community and at the same time fulfills the individual. It is transcendentalism at its best.

"I will grow as nature shall determine," Thoreau writes. This is the natural human we could ourselves become. A person allows their inborn self to emerge, step by step, often haltingly. The natural human is not necessarily the person who spends time in the woods and on mountains, but one who allows life to shape them in the face of any intentions they may have. They are not in nature or part of nature; they are natural themselves. Their plan is not as important as the narrative that emerges gradually from the life in them. They are receptive and cooperative and usually not in control.

I could never have predicted my life's course, it took so many unexpected turns. Yet I can see from this vantage point how one episode led to another and then to another, until I ended up exactly where I would have wanted to be. I have a good marriage, wondrous children, and amazing work. I did not plan any of it, and I never could have expected it. The only "secret" I have about it is that I was willing, probably too innocently, to make big changes whenever the willow fluttered. Friends advised me against many of my choices, because those decisions were not always wise. But mine was the way of the holy fool, and it appears that Henry David Thoreau was also a holy fool, trusting in life and in the quirky inner guide that led him to Walden Pond and beyond. As we reflect on his life and philosophy, we might keep in mind his celebrated eccentricity.

"I will grow as nature shall determine," Thoreau says. I might put it this way: "I will become the person that life wants me to be." I will watch as the life I become accustomed to gives way to something new. I will learn to hold onto my current life softly, not grasping. I might even expect my present direction to last only a while, until the next turn of the wheel.

"I must not be for myself, but God's work." I heard that kind of pious affirmation many times in my life, but now I hear it somewhat differently. It makes no sense to do things for myself or according to my own plans, because life is essentially driven by another will, a different plan. I do not want to say much about who or what controls that plan. Maybe it can only be seen in reverse, after the fact, toward the end of life. I look back on my years, and only now can I glimpse the shape and direction of it. When I was living it, I did not know where I was headed.

Part of this approach asks you not to demand too much and not to be rigid in your expectations. If goals are not reached and efforts are spoiled, you might have to reset your future. Everything depends on how you deal with losses and failures. It is useless to pout or even get angry. It is certainly useless to blame somebody, even yourself. If anything is to blame, it is, as Thoreau says, the breeze. The West Wind again, also known as the Holy Spirit.

The world today puts its trust in facts and machinery. It dispenses with revelation, oracle, poetics, dream, ritual, and inspiration. With its cold, carefully measured, neurotically proven facts, it tries to make a world for humans, but it fails seriously. By disregarding the deepest in human life, the very soul of humanity, it creates both a physical world and a human race that has no interiority and no "miracle," as Ralph Waldo Emerson would say. Whatever it produces has no beating heart, except at times when a soul sneaks into some modern invention. In such a world, people see one person's life as a string of cold events created by personal choices.

In a world where poets can rarely make a living, we see our lives as a quantifiable calendar of facts. I'm not saying that someone, like a master planner in the sky, has it all written down, all planned out. I am just looking at the phenomena, my life story, and seeing it unfolding eerily detailed and directed. It all makes sense, in the end, as though I were following a script.

If this reflection of life events is accurate, then it has some implications. I may become good at reading the signs, at noticing inner promptings and inhibitions, and at following inner guidance. I may seek out not only another will but other intentions for my life. I will know which urges to follow and which to distrust. I will become skilled at listening for hints of where to go and what to do.

I receive my life as passively as the willow leaf that quivers on the brook. We are not talking about being blown by hurricane winds but about fluttering in a soft wind. Emily Dickinson must have been similarly inspired when she wrote:

> In the name of the Bee—
> And of the Butterfly—
> And of the Breeze—Amen![2]

To me, Thoreau's "willow leaf that flutters over the brook" is one of the great images in literature for how to live. Rather than battle through life like a hero, it might be better to flutter over the brook, an age-old image for the flow of life. You stay close to the stream of vitality you sense within you and to the torrent of life that is around you. But you do not go with weapons drawn or tools at hand. You are not a hero with a thousand faces; you are a leaf with dozens of flutters. You don't battle, you tremble, showing that you are alive and close to the source.

3

ETHEREALIZED BY A MOUNTAIN

I go to Flint's Pond for the sake of the mountain view from the hill beyond, looking over Concord. I have thought it the best, especially in the winter, which I can get in this neighborhood. It is worth the while to see the mountains in the horizon once a day. I have thus seen some earth which corresponds to my least earthly and trivial, to my most heavenward-looking, thoughts. The earth seen through an azure, an ethereal, veil. They are the natural temples, elevated brows, of the earth, looking at which, the thoughts of the beholder are naturally elevated and sublimed,—etherealized. I wish to see the earth through the medium of much air or heaven, for there is no paint like the air. Mountains thus seen are worthy of worship.[1]

—Henry David Thoreau, journal entry,
September 12, 1851

A mountain may be a beautiful sight, but if you look at it closely and patiently, it will become part of you, and you will take its meaning into yourself, and you may find a route up out of unconsciousness. You may become more heavenward-looking and develop a vision for your life and ever higher values.

We all live in the dark in some areas, ignorant of our deepest motives and limited in our potentiality—limited, too, by the unconsciousness and dim horizons of the era. But unconsciousness means that you do things without thinking, by habit or custom. Then you are not fully involved and may do things that hurt others or diminish society. Henry David Thoreau's lofty thoughts led him to spend a night in jail to raise consciousness about being a free individual in an encompassing community. His example came to be known as civil disobedience, a dramatic way to advance a society.

A mountain—a natural symbol, in need of no glossary or dictionary of symbols—reminds you of your capacity for transcendence. You know well that you are earthly, but you may forget to rise upward and become ethereal. You may overlook your own ideals and values. Look at a mountain from below and you may learn to live your daily life, active and engaged, while keeping ideals. Occasionally, you do something truly elevated, like going to jail on principle, and you are reminded that you are a mountain.

Interestingly, in another passage Thoreau suggests that when you climb a mountain, you should not rush for the peak but take your time and enjoy the ascent. Remain within the mountain and notice how this aspect of it affects you. Rising gradually is as important as enjoying the summit. In daily life it may be as important to be moving upward as reaching an elevated goal.

I often think of church steeples as having the effect of mountains. When you look at a steeple, your eyes are directed from the broad and solid base to a vanishing point high in the sky. Recently I found myself walking the downtown streets of Charleston, South Carolina, on a hot August day, noticing the many narrow, dark-shingled steeples everywhere around me. Like anorexic mountains, straining toward the sky, they pointed to etherealized life. These stunning needle-like towers, appropriate fixtures on churches, which have high aspirations, could offer me, I felt, celestial thoughts, moral ideals, and nearness to the mysteries. But at that moment I also thought I might remain on the street observing the steeples rather than going into the churches. I felt that the message was more about life than belief.

A natural symbol works on you without any explanation. It takes your mind to a vanishing point, toward thoughts of good effort, success, and vision. Tall steeples can help you get away from whatever is too mundane and pedestrian. I suggest going to the mountains but also appreciating the church steeples in your town. If you want to keep your guiding ideas and high values, you may need to be reminded how far your thoughts need to rise.

It is too easy to become preoccupied with lower concerns, as you focus on making money and buying things and comparing yourself to others and having enough channels of entertainment. You go to the site of a mountain to reset your perspective and rediscover your ascending self. Gradually, you hike out of the lower land of busyness and sense the freedom a mountain can evoke. You want to be better than you have been, and the sight of the mountain reminds you of your higher calling.

Thoreau is not theoretical, telling you that you have a higher nature; he wants to inspire you to have the experience of high places and in that way find out what you are made of. You look at a mountain and say to yourself, *Tat Tvam Asi* (you are that), the teaching of the Upanishads, with which Thoreau was familiar. You become the mountain, knowing your own trails and peaks. A mountain yourself, you poke into the air. Through a natural symbol you find your higher nature.

A nearby mountain can help you become elevated and sublimed, etherealized. From the mountain you could look and see more of the world than usual, your horizons much expanded and your outlook more informed and visionary. From mountain consciousness you find out who your neighbors are and in what ways they are worthy of your attention and emulation. You also find out what is beyond the neighborhood.

My work lies within the perimeters of depth psychology, and usually I recommend going deep into experience and down into dream. Going up often feels like the wrong direction. But the passage from Thoreau about mountain views adds a dimension. You can have higher thoughts without abandoning your appreciation for the depths.

In my life and work I have always paid attention to both depth psychology and religion studies, both soul and spirit. While teaching psychotherapists for many years, I have encouraged them to pay attention to the spiritual lives of their clients and even to include some sort of spiritual direction in their work. I recommend that they study sacred texts of the world and become familiar with concerns of the spirit. You cannot truly care for a person's soul without giving attention to the spirit, just as you should not walk through life without looking at mountains.

On the other hand, my rule is a simple one: You cannot enjoy a thriving spiritual life without giving equal attention to the soul, which is often found in the more ordinary realm of everyday living, even in what Thoreau calls "the ravine." Spiritual work needs grounding in the deeper soul. Otherwise, your focus on the mountain distracts you from life in the world. You may become overly idealistic and drastically moralistic. The soul keeps your vision horizontal and maintains your humanity.

Church steeples are beautiful but also dangerous. Turned sidewise, they look like weapons. On reflection, I found Charleston's dark steeples ominous as well as beautiful. I cannot forget that the Ten Commandments were delivered from a mountaintop. They can offer basic values, but they also have the potential to obscure our humanity and love of life.

Once, I was giving a talk in a church in San Francisco with the Jungian analyst Marion Woodman. We were both speaking from the same pulpit, using one microphone. I enjoyed that comradeship, but it was unusual. Across from us in the sanctuary, the church leaders had placed a steeple. I don't remember why it was there, but I found it unsettling—a huge outdoor image of transcendence within the small inner space of the sanctuary. I learned something about steeples and about transcendence: When they are too close, they can be disturbing and give a mixed, troublesome message. You need a special skill to keep the mountain and the ravine in sight and harmonious.

4

INORGANIC AND LUMPISH

The week I go away to lecture, however much I may get for it, is unspeakably cheapened. The preceding and succeeding days are a mere sloping down and up from it.

In the society of many men, or in the midst of what is called success, I find my life of no account, and my spirits rapidly fall . . . I would rather hear a single shrub oak leaf at the end of a wintry glade rustle of its own accord at my approach, than receive a shipload of stars and garters from the strange kings and people of the earth.

By poverty, i. e. simplicity of life and fewness of incidents, I am solidified and crystalized, as a vapor or liquid by cold. It is a singular concentration of strength and energy and flavor.

Chastity is perpetual acquaintance with the All.

You think that I am impoverishing myself by withdrawing from men, but in my solitude I have woven for myself a silken web or crysalis, and, nymph-like, shall erelong burst forth a more perfect creature, fitted for a higher society. By simplicity, com-

monly called poverty, my life is concentrated and so becomes organized, or a cosmos, which before was inorganic and lumpish.[1]

—Henry David Thoreau, journal entry, February 8, 1857

In this remarkable passage, Henry David Thoreau reveals what for him are the benefits of solitude, keeping a distance from society, and being unmarried. It depends if you want to take the word *chastity* in its usual meaning of purity and the unmarried state, or not being intimately engaged with the world. From a positive point of view, celibacy is "perpetual acquaintance with the All," directing attention away from the world and its concerns and, instead, focusing on higher, absolute values.

Thoreau was a natural monk, not someone dedicated to a religious institution but to nature. For him, poverty could be the way of simplicity. When I was a monk, I, too, took a vow of poverty, not doing without necessities but sharing possessions to foster a spirit of community. Thoreau follows a similar life plan where the sense of commons, the sharing of resources, is deep and intentional.

Sometimes people look for psychological and pathological reasons for Emily Dickinson and Henry David Thoreau finding joy in solitude. Thoreau grasped what for millennia monks have known, that paying close attention to your lifestyle and habits can enhance your spirituality and make your life more meaningful. It is not so much what you believe as how you live. Designing your life consciously is an initial stage in creating a meaningful, spiritual existence. When I was a monk, the lifestyle was at least as important as my thoughts about it. We are back at Thoreau's crucial statement when he left Concord for Walden Pond: "I wished to live deliberately, to front only the essential facts of life."[2]

Thoreau is not impoverished by his solitude. He weaves a "silken web," a chrysalis from which he can emerge as a "perfected creature." He had used this image before, imagining himself a butterfly in embryo, sealed off from the world but in hope of being released and soaring among the best of humanity. It is a good image for anyone, to see your lifestyle as a cocoon in which your potential unfolds.

Thoreau noted that he remained longer in the cocoon, becoming a mature person, than he had expected. But he also said, "I am struck by the fact that the more slowly trees grow at first, the sounder they are at the core, and I think that the same is true of human beings."[3] In a way, he never did grow old, dying at forty-four, and yet he was astonishingly mature in his twenties. He did not look mature to those around him, including Emerson, but he quickly became a striking individual, thoughtful and dedicated to his path.

All of us need appreciation for and patience with ourselves, with little judgment. This is what I get from Thoreau's constant self-effacement: Not neurotic doubt, but a reluctant epiphany, a slow and dubious revelation of self to the world. This hesitant willingness to shine can lead to leadership and boldness that include a dose of doubt, a holding back that can complexify the ultimate appearance of a self that is bold and challenging. His writing, too, gathers strength from his unwillingness to shine too brightly. You can understand his self-defacement as an instrument of his celibacy, being slow to give himself to society and not being forward in his relationships with women.

Thoreau also finds more pleasure in a simple event in nature than in receiving rewards from wealthy and powerful people. This is an important lesson in Thoreau's microethics, his subtle revision of values in which a sum of small new principles eventually accounts for a new way of life. Instead of blindly submitting to a culture of consumerism, he "owned" nature's beauties and mysteries.

The solution to the craving for possessions is not to stifle it, but to transfer it to nature and art, there to be embraced. Instead of going to a big box store to buy an object that has stimulated your craving, go into a forest or park, hungry for the natural world displaying itself. You will not be surprised at the store, but nature will startle you and offer you new discoveries. The gift of nature will satisfy more than the expected thrill of a new possession, which may succumb quickly to buyer's remorse and soon fade away. You bring things into your house and hold onto them, but in nature you encounter potent displays of layered richness.

Thoreau says that the discovery of natural beauty "is a singular concentration of strength and energy and flavor." Possessions tend to rip us apart into many enthusiasms outside ourselves, whereas natural beauty consolidates us and condenses our sense of self. Owning many things that we have gathered unconsciously around us makes us a little mad. First, we crave the thing, and then it becomes too familiar. Our emotions are mixed, uncertain, and scattered.

We could learn to find lasting pleasure in the things of the world. Being at the ocean can provide the sense of awe and wonder necessary for a full human existence. Walking in a forest can offer self-discovery and purpose. Compare a new computer with a nearby rushing stream that offers the sight and sound of vitality. We could live daily with simple desire instead of compulsion. We could be consolidated people instead of the hosts of scattered emotions.

According to Thoreau, when we have found a way to be among things, we will find ourselves more organized and organic in a concentrated cosmos. The word *cosmos* refers to the beautiful order of the world. A cosmos is an organic realm, beautiful for its natural composition and harmonious manifestation. It is not lumpish, having parts sticking out madly all over.

Consider your own cosmos, the way in which you are a world. Are you lumpish, or do you have an organic composition? Do your cravings pull you out and away from your base, or do your desires organize your life? Does your relationship to the world crystalize you, like water turning to ice?

Thoreau describes self-limiting as the condensing power of chastity and poverty. By restricting your association with society, you strengthen your connection to the All. You are less distracted and pulled apart. You are not alone or a loner, but your need for friendship finds satisfaction in a mystic way rather than in social activities.

When I lived under the vows of poverty, chastity, and obedience, these ideals gave me focus, and I have never been richer deep inside myself or clearer about who I am. I was not wandering through life but instead guided by strong values. These vows represented a withdrawal from society, a distancing from the standard way to live. At the same time, we monks were consciously displaying a model for society of an unusually focused way of life. We demonstrated that toning down the need for possessions and romantic partnerships made community more real and felt.

Thoreau equates poverty with simplicity, which organizes the self and gives it a smooth shape. It offers beauty of form, where nothing is out of place, nothing awkward. In his simplicity, Thoreau was not depriving himself but polishing his life and shaping it. Plotinus, the great philosopher of soul, said that our task as humans is to sculpt our souls, chipping away here and carving out there. This is a kind of poverty: simplifying, chipping away, letting go of whatever does not fit. Its goal is a beautiful form where nothing is exaggerated or out of place, nothing lumpish.

5

THE SOUND OF THE ROOSTER

Above all, we cannot afford not to live in the present. He is blessed over all mortals who loses no moment of the passing life in remembering the past. Unless our philosophy hears the cock crows in every barn-yard within our horizon, it is belated. That sound commonly reminds us that we are growing rusty and antique in our employments and habits of thought. His philosophy comes down to a more recent time than ours. There is something suggested by it not in Plato nor the New Testament. It is a newer testament,—the gospel according to this moment. He has not fallen astern; he has got up early, and kept up early and to be where he is is to be in season, in the foremost rank of time. It is an expression of the health and soundness of Nature, a brag for all the world,—healthiness as of a spring burst forth, a new fountain of the Muses, to celebrate this last instant of time. Where he lives no fugitive slave laws are passed. Who has not betrayed his master many times since last he heard that note?[1]

—Henry David Thoreau, "Walking"

Toward the end of his classic essay on walking, Henry David Thoreau devotes a paragraph to the uses of time. When he writes, "we cannot afford not to live in the present," I do not think he is foreshadowing what would be said in our time, the admonition to be in the moment. In that wording we romanticize time and think of nothing but the few fleeting seconds at hand. Live in the present, we are told.

But time is not that simple. We must always contend with the past and think about the future. Both affect the way we are in the present. If we do not have them in mind, our present may be vacant, experimental, and simply improvisatory. If I didn't have the past much in mind, I couldn't put together a book of this nineteenth-century writer and reflect on his words, and yet I would like to make him current. As you read, I hope you hear a rooster crowing.

Thoreau's reference to the rooster makes it clear that he is talking about not living in the past but being open to a new reality that is rising like the sun and causes the rooster to crow. Thoreau could just as well cite the Greek philosopher Herakleitos saying, "The sun is new each day."

We can be awake to the world in which we live today and not lost in wishes for a golden age. The rooster announces a new day, reminding us that we cannot live the way things were, drifting unconsciously in a dreamlike past. The rooster crows at dawn, a time that is fresh and unknown, a carte blanche on which we can write our own narratives.

Some people maintain the values and habits of their families or follow slogans and ideas they picked up as children and are now outmoded. They have not heard the rooster and need "the gospel according to this moment," so they are locked in someone else's response to the reality of their time. We can learn from Plato without becoming a Platonist. We can appreciate Carl Jung and Sigmund Freud's profound wisdom, but we cannot be a Jungian or Freudian without abusing the time we have. You wake up to this day, to your own life, in a world that has never been seen before.

Living in this moment is equivalent to saying, live your own life, not someone else's. Is this not the primary focus of Thoreau's vernacular lifestyle? He does not live someone else's life or occupy someone else's portal of time. He asks, What am I to do? What does my time ask of me? A mere fourteen years younger than the great man, he is not even in Ralph Waldo Emerson's time. If you are going to live in the present, you face the challenges of your specific time frame. Emerson's time was too late for Thoreau. He benefitted from the friendship and the passing on of knowledge, but he could not find his own way in Emerson's wake. They might have got along better if they both had read and understood this passage from "Walking."

You can also be present and awake when the spring of the Muses gushes and you find your way and your inspiration. It does not do to be inspired too late, to find yourself in a cultural milieu that has already spent itself. You are driven by the events and developments of your time, just as Thoreau shaped his life by the press of abolition and the arrival of the Industrial Revolution in Concord, Massachusetts. You respond to the issues of your era and develop appropriate ideas and strategies.

The potency of Thoreau's voice today, over two hundred years after his short walk to Walden Pond, is due as much to the timing of his act as to its content. He was sharply open to the developing life around him and responded. He was not anxiously deciding which religious institution was right for him, he was looking for a religion that would not look like religion, one that was relevant when he awoke in the morning at the edge of a lake and amid trees and animals. He was not going to set himself afire to challenge the official culture of his town, but rather spend a quiet, friendly night in jail to protest a small tax that even his jailer offered to pay. Some people scoff when they learn that Thoreau spent only one comfortable night in jail. They don't understand that it is the ritual of the act that is important and that speaks to generations. Thoreau heard the rooster and came up with an original plan.

We might also understand Thoreau's frequent harping about the citizens of Concord and their annoying habits as chiding them to wake up to a new situation, to the ugliness of slavery and the deadening effect of conventional religion. For himself, he was driven to find a lifestyle and life work suited to him.

Thoreau's artistic genius—which allowed him to formulate his choices into a loosely packed, largely practical philosophy of life, presented in quaint but inspired sentences with local references and penetrating insights—gives him his relevance today and his staying power. He was strictly of his time, dedicated to it, and that is why, paradoxically, his words are timeless. When you attend to the rooster who marks your own time, you discover your destiny, and your life work follows.

Others of our time inspire us—say, a Martin Luther King Jr.—who understood how to surrender himself precisely to his time. But King was of my time and my world. Younger people today did not have him in their present, as I did in mine. I feel blessed. His words are still sounding in my memory, and I can hear them and act on them. For many people today, he is a voice in history, outside of the present.

Thoreau's injunction to live in the moment is not about allowing the world to penetrate your senses second by second, clear of all other considerations. It is about responding to your world and not hiding defensively in the issues of another cultural era or in some manufactured quality of timelessness. It is about hearing the rooster and waking up early in your cosmos and finding solutions to your chink of history. Waking to the dawn of your existence, you are ready, now, to make your mark.

6

THE SACRED SWAMP

Life consists with wildness. The most alive is the wildest . . . My spirits infallibly rise in proportion to the outward dreariness. Give me the ocean, the desert, or the wilderness . . . When I would recreate myself, I seek the darkest wood, the thickest and most interminable, and to the citizen, the most dismal swamp. I enter a swamp as a sacred space—a sanctum sanctorum. There is the strength, the marrow of Nature. The wild-wood covers the virgin mould—and the same soil is good for men and for trees. A man's health requires as many acres of meadow to his prospect as his farm does loads of muck. These are the strong meats on which he feeds. A town is saved, not more by the righteous men in it than by the woods and swamps that surround it. A township where one primitive forest waves above, while another primitive forest rots below,—such a town is fitted to raise not only corn and potatoes, but poets and philosophers for the coming ages.[1]

—Henry David Thoreau, "Walking"

Thoreau is happiest when he is in a dismal place. In this he is like Marquis de Sade, another outlier and curmudgeon who was a gadfly to his neighbors. The marquis had an outrageous, inborn taste for everything that polite society abhorred. He preferred the darkest and most vile situations and found meaning and joy in them. Similarly, but not nearly so extreme, Thoreau seems to have had a natural inclination away from proper society toward the slimier and muddier aspects of nature. He does not cultivate orchids, but likes to sink his feet in the muck of swamps and the sandy shallows of rivers.

A brief comparison of these two passionate writers, Marquis de Sade and Henry David Thoreau, might offer some insight into Thoreau. Perhaps he was not so much against mannered society, which he might dismiss as fussy, but dedicated to his peculiar pleasures, which had everything to do with mud and dirt. In de Sade's case, it took a certain brood of philosophers and artists to see the value of his dark point of view, the explicit sexual and violent scenes he created. Surrealists especially were interested in de Sade's perverted vision, and in my role as a depth psychologist, I found profound insights in his writings.

Similarly, a psychotherapist like me might be drawn to Thoreau, the man of the muddy waters and stinky swamps. It is my job to listen to the messy tales of clients who need to unburden themselves of rotting memories and unsavory situations. My type tends to be interested in the dark side of human nature, not enjoying the acting out but having an interest in what makes human beings act the way they do. In de Sade, it is the sexual oddities, the quirky points of view, the pleasure taken in giving abuse, and especially enjoying the private parts of the human body—all taken metaphors for the slimy side of the psyche. In Thoreau, it is his love of the swamp and all that is muddy and soiling, his resistance to beautifying too much his beloved nature and his natural way of life.

It is not the human body that concerns Thoreau, but the body of the world, nature in all its particulars. He wants to be close to nature as it is, not romanticized or sentimentalized. The dirtier, the better. To make his point clearly, he says that the dismal swamp gets him excited and helps him in his work of finding out who he is *essentially*. Ordinary people, too, often discover the mystery of who they are through their more shameful thoughts and actions.

Thoreau used the telling word *essential* in the famous lines from *Walden* about his experiment at the pond: "I went to the woods because I wished to live deliberately, to front only the essential facts of life." Marquis de Sade felt that the sentimental philosophies of normal society offer only a partial view of the human experience, leaving out the primitive and savage urges of ordinary people. He thought it was his given task to reveal those omissions. Thoreau, too, is willing to be an outcast and a misunderstood neighbor by presenting his unusual thoughts and his rough tastes in his way of life and his writing. He does this work by "fronting the essentials" of his own existence and allowing a philosophy to unfold from that steady and determined engagement with raw life.

Here is a clue to making the world a better place: You focus on the essentials and do not get lost in the nonessentials. You find out from nature what is raw and from human society what is cooked. Habitually you go for the raw, in many senses of the word—essential, unrefined, pioneer, experimental, naked, natural, and crude. Each of these words could be applied to Thoreau. You live the mythology of Eden, encountering the world as if for the first time in a garden from whose clay the first man was made.

You can gain valuable insights through study and reading, but the raw encounter with the world comes first. Otherwise, you are biased and shielded when you first notice the arrival of spring or first scan the landscape from a mountain. Much of contemporary experience is secondary and derivative. We have seen the movie or read the book. There is little primary discovery in modern life. Rather than remain for a moment in glorious ignorance, today we rush to an encyclopedia of knowledge on our handy electronic devices, which can serve as apotropaic, danger shields protecting us from the very rawness Thoreau appreciates.

A middle-aged man writes to me saying that he loves his wife, but he has a friend, a woman he has known for years, who suddenly causes his heart to flutter. He phones me and says, "Help me deal with this. It is too complicated for me. I don't know how to handle it." At first, I think of suggestions I could give him, but then a Thoreau thought flashes into my mind. This is life. Complex and beautiful in its own way. An appearance of eros, which is never clear and predictable. I suggest that he trust himself, stay close to all that he loves, stay in the muck of it and work it out.

Therapists can stand in the way of pristine experience, and experts can take away the frisson of original discovery that makes life passionate. It is no wonder that many people find contemporary life depressing: We are afraid of original experiences and essential human conundrums. We are happy to take a pill to eradicate bothersome challenges or create a sanitized existence in which there are no emotional swamps.

Thoreau goes into nature to find wildness, the wild potential he has within him, that aspect of himself that he doesn't know and understand. Thoreau chooses to be raw naturally rather than to participate in the elaborate defensive concoctions of society. He prefers to listen to crickets than to go to the opera.

It would help us all to reflect on what it means to be wild. It may not be as literal and as physical as growing your hair out and living in the forest. After all, at Walden Pond, Thoreau built a cabin, which he insisted on calling a house. He lived only two miles from town and from the family home, where his mother and sister lived. He walked to town regularly and ate his mother's food either in his lake house or often, very often, in town. He was moderate in his wildness, or you could say that simultaneously he was able to live two lives: one in nature and one in town. These choices help define what he means by wildness and how to live originally.

Here is yet another guideline for us: Let us opt out of the superficiality of modern life and remain in touch with the swamps and ravines. A town needs inspiring forests waving above and frightening forests rotting below. The last clarifying line from this important passage must be quoted as Thoreau wrote it, and it needs no commentary: "Such a town is fitted to raise not only corn and potatoes, but poets and philosophers for the coming ages."

7

A DOSE OF MYSELF

When I am invited to lecture anywhere,—for I have had a little experience in that business,—that there is a desire to hear what I think on some subject, though I may be the greatest fool in the country,—and not that I should say pleasant things merely, or such as the audience will assent to; and I resolve, accordingly, that I will give them a strong dose of myself. They have sent for me, and engaged to pay for me, and I am determined that they shall have me, though I bore them beyond all precedent.

So now I would say some thing similar to you, my readers. Since you are my readers, and I have not been much of a traveller, I will not talk about people a thousand miles off, but come as near home as I can. As the time is short, I will leave out all the flattery, and retain all the criticism.[1]

—Henry David Thoreau, "Life Without Principle"

Having spent thirty years traveling to give lectures at all kinds of venues in countless places, I know a little about the situation Thoreau is describing. Much of the time I have felt inadequate, knowing the limitations of my knowledge and especially my ability to excite my audiences and give them what they need and want. I have sat in green rooms, contemplating the talk I am about to give, trying to push aside the gaps in my abilities. I have told myself to simply give them who and what I am. If that is not enough, I should hang up my speaker's jacket and try some other line of work.

The principle holds for all interactions. Sitting with a client in psychotherapy, consulting at a hospital, or teaching at a university—I am inadequate, as everyone is, even if they don't know it. All I can do is give my clients a dose of myself and hope that is sufficient. I never drown in my shortcomings or offer weak leadership and counsel, but an interior voice always reminds me where I come from.

Like Thoreau, I know that I am a little rough around the edges. To ease any tension, I usually remind my audience that I am the son of a plumber. I was the first in my family to go to college, and as a young man I never watched anyone I knew stand in front of a large crowd and tell them things that they might take to heart and treasure.

My readers and attendees tell me they like to hear the stories of my life, and in that I am also close to Thoreau. His audiences pleaded with him to skip over the theory and talk about his life. I tell them of events "as near home as I can." I am not much of a traveler, so I cannot describe far-off exotic places. I can only talk about my limited life and be myself.

Thoreau is afraid that if he offers himself to his audience, he will appear as a fool. Certainly, to give yourself over to the world could be foolish because we all know how imperfect we are, with so much raw material to work out and so much to learn. I know that in my own lecturing, in those moments when I want to be vulnerable to my audience, I am taking a risk. I have also learned that, for a variety of reasons, people in an audience may wish that the speaker or leader fail. They may find some pleasure in witnessing a successful person or merely someone in a higher position "come down to their level."

I have often asked myself, should I offer what I expect the audience will accept and appreciate, or should I give them myself, a more complex and challenging message? Should I look for safety in presenting familiar and unchallenging thoughts, or should I speak my truth? Almost always I opt for the fool's way and say what is important to me. I notice that often it isn't what people want to hear, and when they talk to me after a presentation they suggest that I read an author they like, often one that either I know personally or one I do not regard highly. Sometimes they press a book into my hand by an author I do not hold dear.

Once, I got involved in an organization that I hoped would help me improve my presentations and make me more successful. I spent over a year giving talks in their style, not mine. On one occasion, I was in another country, where a friend brought her husband to hear me. I knew it was a sensitive moment for them. But I didn't bring myself and gave someone else's idea of a good talk. With every word I uttered, I could tell that my usual quality was lost, and I felt that I had betrayed my friend. After that painful experience, I gave up my fool's errand and went back to trusting my own methods. The way to personal strength is simply being there, showing up with a willingness to reveal yourself.

If you are going to show up, come with your home territory, too. Do not pretend to be from somewhere else, but speak your own language and dialect, and infuse the moment with the wisdom of your native place. Be a particular human being with your own place of origin with all its advantages and its peculiarities. Be vernacular. Do not borrow a more exalted language or exotic references.

Having the plumber spirit in me, I bring with me the earthiness of trades workers who are my people. Sometimes I am told that it is marvelous that I can take complicated ideas and make them understandable. Well, I am sorry, but that is all I can do. My roots lie in the world of water closets and waste management. I can only speak adequately to plumbers and their ilk. You think I am cleverly reducing rich ideas to something the ordinary person can understand, but the truth is, speaking the vernacular is the best I can do.

Thoreau says that he is a clodhopper and cannot do any better. The same with me. I am a plumber's son. Thoreau says that if you want to meet him, you will be disappointed when you do. It is the same with me. I am a plumber's son. I can't do any better. You will be disappointed.

But let me tell you. If there was ever a PhD in plumbing, it should have been granted to my father. He quit school in the tenth grade and went on to work with doctoral engineers who sought out his advice. A well-regarded psychiatrist came to him every two weeks, for a period, to talk over his cases.

Thoreau was a PhD clodhopper, and that is the secret to his place in world culture. If you grasp this clue about his existence, you will know how to read his natural mysticism and appreciate his carefully crafted writing style. He remained loyal to the lowliness of his calling even as he explored the heights.

Not only in lectures but in all his encounters, Thoreau showed people who he was and where he came from and let the chips fall. Sometimes this approach got him in trouble, as when he had to wait years to have his writing published or when he did not receive the invitation to speak that he hoped for. Or possibly when the love of his life turned down his proposal and married someone else. In the end, this personal philosophy led to the creation of Henry David Thoreau, a force in human history.

We could all be "made" in this way. Just as Henry became Thoreau, the figure so many admire and emulate, each of us could become someone. Someone! The perfection of who we were from day one. That is the point and the goal. To give the world a strong picture of who you are. Ultimately, simply to be, the ultimate root of personal power.

As to his appearance, Emerson wrote: "He was of short stature, firmly built, of light complexion, with strong, serious blue eyes and a grave aspect." A man named Willis, who knew him in his youth, remembering him forty years later, said he was tall and straight. Even today, Thoreau's stature seems to be in the eye of the beholder.

The ultimate secret is to show the world who you are. Let your being shine. Be the person you know well and who may be embarrassing to you. Be vernacular in your own territory. Speak your own language. Use your own metaphors. Tell your own stories. Love the local self you are and make it a gift to whoever is listening.

8

ACCIDENTS

There is always some accident in the best things, whether thoughts or expressions or deeds. The memorable thought, the happy expression, the admirable deed are only partly ours. The thought came to us because we were in a fit mood; also we were unconscious and did not know that we had said or done a good thing. We must walk consciously only part way toward our goal, and then leap in the dark to our success. What we do best or most perfectly is what we have most thoroughly learned by the longest practice, and at length it falls from us without our notice as a leaf from a tree. It is the last time we shall do it,—our unconscious leavings.[1]

—Henry David Thoreau, journal entry, March 11, 1859

The word *accident* comes from a root that means "fall," and accidents do fall into your life unexpectedly. In my early thirties I considered cautiously whether I should attend the Syracuse University doctoral program in religion. My own ideas about religion even then were radical and unconventional. I did not know if I should take the risk of going through the rigors of a doctoral education at a university unknown to me. I almost backed out.

At Syracuse, not only did I receive an excellent education, I made lifelong friends with people who were also my teachers: James Wiggins, David L. Miller, and Huston Smith. I also met James Hillman, who became one of my closest friends and important influences. I was looking for deep learning, and Hillman came into my life accidentally, an unexpected gift. I went to Syracuse not knowing if it was the best choice and kept leaping into the dark. Today, I don't think I could do the work that has given my life meaning if I had not answered the invitation to that extraordinary university.

Something inspired Hillman, who was living in Europe at the time, to send me offprints of articles he was publishing in obscure journals. Those clippings, which I now keep on a bookshelf over my shoulder as I write, gave me a direction for my life work. They would arrive unexpectedly in my mailbox at Syracuse and change the way I thought and lived. I attended Syracuse for their good faculty; when Hillman showed up, it was an accident.

Seeing an accident as "part of" a good conscious effort is the key element in Thoreau's insightful idea about how thoughts and projects develop. We may be so absorbed in our intentions and efforts that we do not realize the importance of unexpected appearances of fresh material and new people. Thoreau suggests that we actively leap into our unconsciousness and let it do its work. We can design a life that allows such accidents to happen.

The Greeks honored a special god for the unexpected: Hermes, a trickster and a thief who represents the tendency of life to take things from us and sometimes to add. Hermes may snatch away your health, a family member, a career, precious objects. But as the god of surprises, he may also leave things for you when you least expect them, like walking into a store and finding money or sitting down in a train and finding a book that was left behind and that changes your life for the good. In ancient times, people also pronounced the name "Hermes" when someone sneezed, a kind of accident. My life has been full of Hermes sneezes.

When I publish a book, I know that Hermes, the god of words and communication, deserves at least half the credit. The writing process is full of accidents, things falling from the sky and making their way into the book: a word that stands out in a conversation, the discovery of a new book, a new play on words. I am on the alert and watch for ideas and language that I would not find by myself. For this, Thoreau says we must find ourselves in a fit mood and at least slightly unconscious. If we are too awake, we may not grasp the accidental material that is often the richest.

James Hillman points out a related Renaissance principle for the artist: "Noticing," a special habit of not overlooking things that catch your eye. You notice a Hermes gift that you could ignore but that might be significant. You need to be unconscious for a while, but you cannot lose your power to notice.

If you have embarked on a project, do not try to accomplish everything yourself. Leave some room for Hermes. Do not think that you are superhuman and can do the whole job. Part of your skill is to know when to pause and allow this fertile spirit into your daily life. You can get to know the ways of Hermes and cooperate with his interventions more effectively.

Thoreau suggests walking partway into your project consciously and then taking a leap into the dark. Inspirations will drop into your lap like leaves falling from a tree. The process is not so much about employing your skills and applying your craft, but getting things started in the right direction and then allowing the rest to happen unaware, which could mean with the aid of the gods. You work your project with one hand using your skill and leave the other open to guidance by an invisible creative force.

The ancient Greeks honored another inspiring agency in life: the Muses, the nine sister goddesses of inspiration. Today we tend to think of a muse as the talent a creative person might have for finding inspiration, or sometimes the muse is found in another person who inspires. But the Greeks treated the Muses as autonomous presences that play a central role in creative work. Personifying and objectifying these powers invite dialogue and collaboration, a form of invisible guidance that is more effective than pure mental effort.

The muse is never seen as a power that does the complete task of a work of art. She can inspire and support. In that way, she is like the helper Thoreau mentions. You go on your own power for a while, and then you let the muse enter the process. Sometimes the muse inspires the work from the beginning, and then you apply your skills. In either case, you share your creative process with a powerful agent that is not you.

Creative unconsciousness can enter a project through long repetition of an action. You develop a habit in your work and eventually can perform a task without thinking about it. Thoreau recommends intentionally including this kind of activity in your work, making it part of your technique. Most modern people want to be alert and in control, but here the idea is to plan for unconsciousness.

I find this approach especially effective in playing the piano. If I can get to a point in memorizing a piece where my fingers do the playing without any interference from my consciousness, I can play the piece securely. I am not committing the music to memory, but rather getting it inserted into my hands and fingers.

Once, the poet David Whyte was sharing a stage with me in London. Together, we each did our own performances. I read from my writings and he recited poetry without any written texts. Afterward, I asked him how he could do this so effectively. He explained that he does not memorize the poems, exactly, but gets to know them so that the recital does not come from memory but from knowing.

As I understand him, there is an element of unconsciousness in his method. He intends it to be part of the process. If he were more conscious, his memory would be a mental operation and probably less secure.

In any case, Thoreau's suggestion is useful; in many situations we could trust our unconscious powers to do the work for us. We could style our activity so it leaves room for other influences. Hermes will still arrive when he wants, but it does not hurt to prepare for his appearance.

9

CONSULT YOUR GENIUS

I find that actual events, notwithstanding the singular prominence which we all allow them, are far less real than the creations of my imagination. They are truly visionary and insignificant—all that we commonly call life & death—and affect me less than my dreams. This petty stream which from time to time swells & carries away the mills and bridges of our habitual life—and that mightier stream or ocean on which we securely float—what makes the difference between them?

Considering how few poetical friendships there are, it is remarkable that so many are married. It would seem as if men yielded too easy an obedience to nature without consulting their genius. One may be drunk with love without being any nearer to finding his mate. There is more of good nature than of good sense at the bottom of most marriages. But the good nature must have the counsel of the good spirit or Intelligence.[1]

—Henry David Thoreau to Harrison Gray Otis Blake, September 23, 1852

In Henry David Thoreau's world, as in ours, people placed higher value on actual events than on fantasy and imagination. By fantasy I do not mean wild ideas and wishes, but the serious images that lie enfolded in all our thoughts and actions. Our decisions and behaviors act out a narrative that may be conscious to us or entirely hidden. How many times do we respond to our partner with the same gestures and language of a parent? How often do we seek a career impelled on the same patterns that our ancestors made sense of life? The past is like a treasury of possibilities from which to choose a present course of action. Often—or always—it is more enlightening to consider the stories and personalities we bring to life, such as the narratives just described, than to sort out actions taken literally.

Thoreau says that matters of life and death affect him less than his dreams. From my therapeutic practice, I am sure that I know a person better from an examination of their dreams than from the things they tell me about themselves. Or I can listen to the stories of their life, as tales and imaginings that change with each telling, and know them well.

I listen to my client's dream and watch stories from life weave in and around it, and I notice how the dream intersects with actual life, elucidating themes and echoes that would be invisible without it. In the end, dreams are more revealing and closer to emotions and meaning than direct explanations. I am surprised to read Thoreau's words and see that he was, among things, an early depth psychologist. Sigmund Freud was born six years before Thoreau died.

Thoreau suggests that we float on an ocean of images and see that in comparison the shallow streams of ordinary life are paltry. The ocean gives us our depth and power, and we gain confidence by floating safely on its currents. In this passage he is clearly recommending that we remain in contact with the ocean of imagination instead of the thin waters of literal, one-dimensional life.

The example he gives is one that most people know intimately. "One may be drunk with love without being any nearer to finding his mate." You may follow your strong emotions into a serious relationship, but then you discover that a union of two people requires experience and an intelligence about the heart. You think your feelings are trustworthy but then discover that they can be illusions. It might be better to float on the greater and deeper ocean of imagination and benefit from its important themes and laws. You may be overwhelmed by desire for another person, but when you get closer you may discover that love is not enough to make a good union. In many marriages there is more good nature than good sense.

People act on their feelings alone without consulting their genius and intelligence. They must think that it is best to act on feelings without first sorting them out. Maybe that is what Thoreau means when he notes how few "poetical" friendships there are and yet many marriages. A poetical friendship is one that is *examined* and *deliberate*, to use the key words Thoreau used to describe his purpose in moving to Walden Pond. He wanted those qualities in his life.

"Poetical" might also refer to the images that underlie daily life, the poetics of daily experience by which we notice the narratives, images, and themes that give life its shape and dynamics. You may notice that you are sad among your untroubled friends, like Hamlet brooding in his castle. You may find that you are persecuted for your efforts to make a better world, like Jesus tortured and cruelly executed. You may feel a longing to find your home, like Odysseus trying to get back to Ithaca. The underlying themes are essential, yet they are sometimes difficult to detect.

These are obvious poetical references in life, but you may also find more subtle ones. In looking for a partner, are you searching for a mother or a lover or a companion? Are memories of past relationships interfering with the current one? These, too, are fantasies and narratives, the poetics of daily experience. They operate as grander themes and images lying beneath your conscious aims. They are part of the ocean that sustains you.

An intelligence in these matters is not analytical or mathematical but a thoughtful quest for depth. A dream may give us a hint as to the dynamics going on in a relationship, or the dream ego's action may show signs of defense, fear, and avoidance. Examining past relationships or marriages of friends and family members could reveal patterns that are at work in the present but are hidden. It is odd that the essentials are usually the most undetectable.

Thoreau's advice is not to avoid mistakes in love but to pay attention to the many narratives and themes influencing us from the oceanic depths. This attention to the poetics of life can prepare us to work out the intricacies of love more successfully. They constitute a kind of intelligence that is different from the practical mind we prize so much in our time. It is an intelligence of depth and imagination, not of fact and strategy.

It is difficult for me to understand how this man who was never married and apparently never excelled at human connection could write so meaningfully about love. But his life was intense, and he sorted it out regularly in his journals. He was also a dedicated reader, who knew the classics, Eastern philosophy, and current ideas. He attended and lectured at an active lyceum in his town and traveled, giving talks and engaging with many creative people. Thoreau was especially good at translating the laws of nature into the ways of human life. I'm tempted to think that he learned about marriage from his many journeys in boats and canoes.

Perhaps during his paddles he was exploring the roots and undercurrents of human life. The mountains Thoreau contemplated and climbed taught him lessons in love. The ancient Greeks described Eros as the generative and sustaining power in all of life, the ruler of the cosmos. In that sense Thoreau's close encounters with nature gave him a deep understanding of how humans live and love.

10

DIPPED TOAST

It is a singular infatuation that leads men to become clergymen in regular, or even irregular, standing. I pray to be introduced to new men, at whom I may stop short and taste their peculiar sweetness. But in the clergyman of the most liberal sort I see no perfectly independent human nucleus, but I seem to see some indistinct scheme hovering about, to which he has lent himself, to which he belongs . . . a man's creed can never be written . . . What great interval is there between him who is caught in Africa and made a plantation slave of in the South, and him who is caught in New England and made a Unitarian minister of? In course of time they will abolish the one form of servitude, and, not long after, the other. I do not see the necessity for a man's getting into a hogshead and so narrowing his sphere, not for his putting his head into a halter. Here's a man who can't butter his own bread, and he has just combined with a thousand like him to make a dipped toast for all eternity.[1]

—Henry David Thoreau, journal entry, February 28, 1857

The transcendentalists generally encouraged living your own life and being your own person. "Self-reliance," Ralph Waldo Emerson called it, and William Ellery Channing advised "self-culture—the care which every man owes to himself, to the unfolding and perfecting of his nature." If this was a rule for other transcendentalists, for Henry David Thoreau it was an obsession. He worked all his life to create a way of life that allowed him to be an individual and not a copy of anyone else or anyone's theory. The batter of dipped toast might be, metaphorically, a belief system or a special role in society. He especially disdained the conventionality of townspeople. He left his home in Concord, Massachusetts, to discover the kind of thoughtful, deliberate life that was suited to him.

This rule applied especially to religion. Thoreau preferred to find sanctity in a swim or a view from a mountain to sitting in an uncomfortable, straight, and confined church pew. And so, in this prickly passage he decries the minister who speaks from his beliefs and theological lessons that to Thoreau were like bread dipped in batter.

In our modern world, too, people have a hard time talking to each other when their beliefs and ideologies, covering them like egg dip, prevent them from having a real conversation. You find natural openness in Thoreau's writing style, as well. He forever refers to an experience he had that day or to a local place or personality. For the most part, Thoreau lived locally and presented himself as a person with a local life and personal experience.

We could take a lesson from Thoreau's aim to be vernacular and individual, especially in our time, when we are so deeply influenced by worldwide media that encourage a common language and ideas. We all speak, to some extent, as the media teach us to speak. Our very ideas flow directly from the current source of news and entertainment to our brains and tongues, and so we parrot their ideas as if they were our own.

It takes an effort of attention and practice to speak for ourselves and generally to be real people—to hesitate, at least, when a phrase comes to mind that has leapt directly from the international news program to our lips. We have the choice to consider borrowed thoughts and words and then make them our own. Even some personal editing might help us preserve our individuality where in an instant it might be surrendered to some pronouncement flowing through the opinion outlets. We could avoid becoming dipped toast.

For myself as a writer I am careful not to overdo my sources and speak in someone else's voice. One day my literary agent, who is both an advisor and a friend, told me that with my next book I should not refer so much to Carl Jung and James Hillman. Suddenly, my face turned red. I could feel the embarrassing realization that I had overdone those dear influences. Now I hope I have changed. I do my best to honor them without giving them too much attention. I am trying to reclaim my own ideas and values. To an extent, I go back to who I was before I read their work and speak more from my own inner resource. I was dipping my bread too much in their delicious sauces.

Speaking for yourself is a risk. You could be wrong. If you make a mistake, it is your own doing. You can't blame the person you are quoting or relying on. You dig deep into yourself and find inspiration and wisdom there, not in someone else who has proven to be important and valuable.

A clergyperson often speaks for the broad system and tradition they have adopted and may be hardly discernible as an individual. They are coated in a special beloved topping of teachings and customs. Their language is not their own. Personally, I find it sad to listen to someone, even a layperson, devoted to a religion speak to me in language that comes from their beliefs rather than themselves. Where are *you*?, I wonder, in that mass of memorized citations from a scripture. Do you realize how much you have surrendered of yourself, how you have disappeared in the thick gravy of your beliefs? Is that acceptable to you, or are you pleased with that disappearance? Is it not preferable to work things out on your own and take full responsibility for your worldview, your moral values, and your way of life?

We could study ourselves carefully, all of us, to see whether our beliefs have grown over us and obscured who we are. Have they become a means of disappearing, of escaping the human condition and our own situation? Are our ideologies methods for escaping from ourselves? And is it preferable to be free of the responsibility of living as individuals than to accept the life given to us and work out a best solution for ourselves? Do our beliefs extinguish the self and offer the odd bliss of self-annihilation?

We need a perfectly independent human nucleus, but this essential ingredient is often caught by an enslaver, a snatcher of human souls, who takes away our identity and gives us another that is generic or commercial. Instead of one who thinks for himself, we turn into a Republican or a Democrat, a devotee of the stock market, or a believer in spectator sports. This language is the argot of the pack and not the person. The soul has been put in shackles and is not free to speak for itself.

When we live by ideologies rather than personal intelligence and assessment, the human element goes missing, and naturally we end up in wars and conflicts. Our enemies are not persons, but rather cardboard characters that look like people but have no beating hearts. One political faction hates its opponents because they are not people but toy soldiers in a game. The perception of human individuality might make it more difficult to create easy enemies and indulge in our biases.

Asserting your individuality rather than the various clubs to which you belong might help the world become a more human, more civil, place, where the passions associated with your memberships might be tempered by your personal values. Keep your individual judgment at work and be cautious in joining too generously any social movement that would obscure your individual self, dousing it with an opaque paste.

11

THE CIVILIZED APPLE TREE

Pliny, adopting the distinction of Theophrastus, says, "Of trees there are some which are altogether wild (sylvestres), some more civilized (urbaniores)." Theophrastus includes the apple among the last; and, indeed, it is in this sense the most civilized of all trees. It is as harmless as a dove, as beautiful as a rose, and as valuable as flocks and herds. It has been longer cultivated than any other, and so is more humanized; and who knows but, like the dog, it will at length be no longer traceable to its wild original? It migrates with man, like the dog and horse and cow: first, perchance, from Greece to Italy, thence to England, thence to America; and our Western emigrant is still marching steadily toward the setting sun with the seeds of the apple in his pocket, or perhaps a few young trees strapped to his load. At least a million apple-trees are thus set farther westward this year than any cultivated ones grew last year. Consider how the Blossom-Week, like the Sabbath, is thus annually spreading over the prairies; for when man migrates, he carries with him not only

> *his birds, quadrupeds, insects, vegetables, and his very sward, but his orchard also.*[1]
>
> —Henry David Thoreau, "Wild Apples"

On our small patch of land in rural New Hampshire we have two apple trees that have a more intimate place in our family compared to the oaks, pines, and hemlocks all around. Although one of my favorite pastimes in warm weather is to sit, prop my head up, and contemplate the tall oak crowns swaying in the wind like wildly abandoned Pacific Island dancers, I have more intimate encounters with the apple trees. I notice when limbs cross over each other, or when suckers reach toward the sky instead of cooperating with the other branches to produce fruit. I measure the summer's progress by the size of the apples and look forward to having lunch directly off the trees and tasting tangy homemade cider in the fall.

Henry David Thoreau tells his story of the westward expansion of apple trees, as they become more civilized through their association with humans. But I wonder about the other direction in which the trees humanize us by their friendliness. Thoreau says that the apple tree is as harmless as a dove or a rose, and I see the resemblance. In fact, I feel how the apple trees help me deal with wild emotions. I can almost hear them coo like the mourning doves that sit heavily on the gravel road.

When we first visited the house in which we now live, twelve years ago, we found a building rushed to be completed on land that appeared like a construction site. Now we have dressed the land with soft landscaping and replaced the plastic facade of the house with real materials and altogether created a humanizing environment. The apple trees, now at home in a more civilized setting, seem to reach out to us in friendship. They can be assuring and calming, especially amid the wild forests all around us.

They are not forbidding like noble oaks, and not threatening like massive hemlocks, and not even as imposing as a protective beech. They do not grow as straight or as tall and have many branches and subbranches and subs of those. Carl Jung posted an alchemical image in one of his books showing a stag with a branching rack and a unicorn with a single straight horn. The deer represents the lower, multifaceted soul, he said, and the unicorn is the focused, more militant spirit. I feel that way about the apple tree: It conjures up the soul, while the tall oaks clearly evoke the spirit.

You could say that the soul in general is cozy and the spirit inspiring. The apple tree—low, rich, and sometimes gnarly—tends our humble needs and may offer a feeling of a loved and tended home, especially when it grows close to the house, as ours does. This is a description of humanizing, and so I understand Thoreau saying that the apple tree has civilized the world as it has expanded across national boundaries.

We are talking about the psychological power of plant life in relation to humans. They can convey emotions of calm and belonging, essential qualities for emotional well-being. Continually, by their sheer appearance and natural habits, they relate to us in a healing way that fosters our humanity and stability. We know that about trees in general and about apple trees in particular, but we do not often comment on this extraordinary psychological capacity. We talk about these trees as objects without feeling or relatedness, and yet they become part of the family and have individual relationships with family members.

The fact that apple trees give us a special kind of food also places them in a special relationship with humans because, in a sense, they nourish us and give us sensory pleasure. You can feel the generosity of such a tree, especially when it lives near your home and goes through its own periods of disease and stunted growth and fallowness. When it suddenly comes into health and vigor, it gives you more than ever, and you feel relieved and joyful.

Thoreau was especially charmed by the aroma of an apple. He advised walking down a road lined with apple trees. You get a strong scent of the fruit, a pleasure you do not have to pay for, he says. He also suggested rubbing a handkerchief onto an apple to scent the fabric, instead of using perfumed oils. Two things excite me about these facts. One is that Thoreau understood the importance of scent, an idea that goes back to medieval times, when different aromas were associated with the various planets and used for health. Scenting a cloth with an apple is also another way to employ an apple to civilize humans, one of Thoreau's aims in life.

There are so many things we do not know about trees, apple trees especially. We are beginning to understand how trees are sensitive to their surroundings and to other trees, but we have yet to learn their full range of powers in relation to humans. One day we may know better how they can heal our diseases and relate to us directly. Eventually we may see that Thoreau was a forerunner in seeing how apple trees can humanize us.

You learn from Thoreau's words that he loved, was in love with, apple trees. He said as much about an encounter with a bush: "I felt a positive yearning toward one bush this afternoon. There was a match found for me at last. I fell in love with a shrub oak."[2] I, too, feel a degree of infatuation with our apple trees. Often I sneak a peek at them and feel deeply satisfied to be sharing my life with them, and in some moments it seems that I am enjoying a forbidden infatuation with them. Thoreau might point to a faint echo of Eden there.

12

A BROAD MARGIN TO MY LIFE

I love a broad margin to my life. Sometimes, in a summer morning, having taken my accustomed bath, I sat in my sunny doorway from sunrise till noon, rapt in reverie, amidst the pines and hickories and sumachs, in undisturbed solitude and stillness . . . I grew in those seasons like corn in the night . . . They were not time subtracted from my life, but so much over and above my usual allowance. . . . This was sheer idleness to my follow-townsmen, no doubt, but if the birds and flowers had tried me by their standard, I should not have been found wanting. A man must find his occasions in himself, it is true. The natural day is very calm, and will hardly reprove his indolence.[1]

—Henry David Thoreau, *Walden*

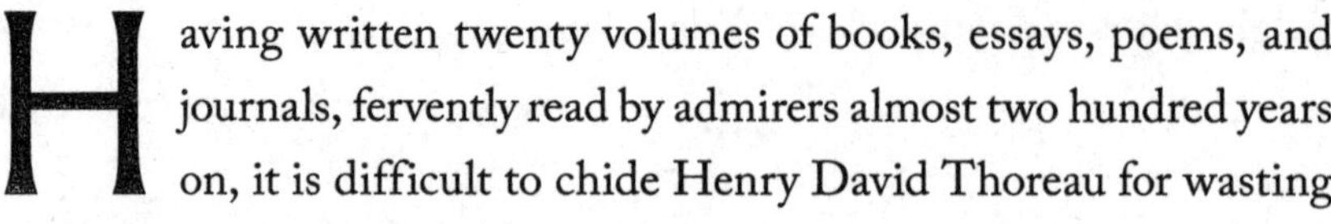

Having written twenty volumes of books, essays, poems, and journals, fervently read by admirers almost two hundred years on, it is difficult to chide Henry David Thoreau for wasting his time. Yet he loved a broad margin to his life, "a halo of ease and leisure," he says elsewhere.[2]

The word *halo* allows us once again to place his comments in the realm of theology and his avowed search for the divine in daily life. There is something sacred about looking for Sabbath among busy days. Sabbath may be sanctified by the tradition of a holy day, such as Sunday, Saturday, Friday, or a special day of the year observed as holy. But it might also be an ordinary day made sacred by giving it an aura of rest.

It is a mistake to think of the margin of leisure as a wasted space in a life otherwise dedicated to worthwhile work. Much can be accomplished in the hours when you do nothing of obvious value. This may be one of the most important lessons for us dealing with an increasingly meaningless world, when you consider that it is also a time dedicated to labor. You are deemed worthless if you don't work effortfully and with supreme dedication. Work is the meaning of your life and the standard by which you are judged as a person.

In these days when we are considering earlier retirement, a shorter work week, more paid time off for family and health, and the coming robots and artificial intelligence, we can be prepared to reimagine the role of work in a noble life. We may all need a wider margin for leisure and a new definition of indolence—another word for laziness.

In conversation I often confess my own kind of creative indolence that is an aspect of my life work: writing. People learn that I have published over thirty books, substantial for the most part, and they say to me: "You must be highly disciplined to get so much done." I feel confused and reply, "Not really. I don't feel disciplined at all. I write for the joy and the pleasure of it."

What I do is not work, but neither is it play. It is a creative activity that fulfills me so deeply and interests me so much that I don't need any self-discipline to get it done. Often, I don't want the writing of a particular book to end, and as soon as it is finished, usually the same day, I start another one. The philosopher Plato said that there are four kinds of divine madness: love, religion, divination, and art. I feel artistic madness in my "work," so that leisure is the background of my labor. I relish the satisfaction of the activity and don't have to go out looking for entertainment.

Doing nothing, the way Thoreau describes it, soothes the soul, eases the heart and body, and stills the mind. When you are not hard at obsessive work, you can get close to nature and see and hear those things that work impedes. You can listen to your thoughts and reflect on what has been happening.

Some people meditate laboriously, trying hard to do it right. They have trouble because what they are doing is not natural. I prefer the advice of a Zen master like Shunryu Suzuki, "The most important thing is to forget all gaining ideas, all dualistic ideas. In other words, just practice zazen in a certain posture. Do not think about anything. Just remain on your cushion without expecting anything. Then eventually you will resume your own true nature. That is to say, your own true nature resumes itself."[3]

I think Thoreau's true nature recovered itself on those mornings when he accomplished nothing in the eyes of the dualistic world, the one that finds doing nothing indolent and doing something, anything, praiseworthy. His "margin of leisure" is Suzuki's zazen, his sitting Suzuki's spiritual practice, his sunny doorway Suzuki's cushion. Persist with doing nothing and in the empty space you will find anything you are looking for because you will have discovered your own nature. That is exactly what Thoreau was searching for with intense devotion. He wanted to know who he was so that he would know for certain what to do.

In those empty times, Thoreau grew "like corn in the night." On a farm, you wake in the morning and the corn is higher than it was yesterday. Much was accomplished during the silence of the dark night. These gaps or margins Thoreau understood and appreciated. In modern life, we have forgotten their potency and importance. We think we should be busy all the time. We forget that when we are sleeping, corn grows.

I have a formula about busyness. People who feel busy look productive, but they are accomplishing little. They *feel* busy, but they are not doing much of worth. Busyness is a psychological complex, a sensation that comes over you when you are visibly active but achieving nothing.

As with any psychological illusion, you can respond by going deeper into your busy life and discover how to work harder. The symptom shows what is needed but doesn't accomplish the work that has to be done. The hectic person eventually might shed the painful, neurotic feeling of being too busy and then really get to work.

Thoreau did not need to justify his existence by working too hard. He saw that the birds and flowers were not busy, but just being themselves. He could sit in his sunny doorway simply "rapt in reverie." Many of us might sit still some day and then make up for lost time by working extra hard later. It would help our society to shed the demanding work ethic and find our margins of pleasure. Our true natures might return and we might finally be calm, and that would be a cure for aggression and violence. The world is in dire need of calm people, people at ease with themselves, people who do not have to work too hard and then resolve their inner conflicts with others. Most of us need a margin of leisure.

13

THE SACRED ART OF FARMING

Ancient poetry and mythology suggest, at least, that husbandry was once a sacred art; but it is pursued with irreverent haste and heedlessness by us, our object being to have large farms and large crops merely. We have no festival, nor procession, nor ceremony, not excepting our Cattle-shows and so called Thanksgivings, by which the farmer expresses a sense of the sacredness of his calling, or is reminded of its sacred origin. It is the premium and the feast which tempt him. He sacrifices not to Ceres and the Terrestrial Jove, but to the infernal Plutus rather. By avarice and selfishness, and a grovelling habit, from which none of us is free, of regarding the soil as property, or the means of acquiring property chiefly, the landscape is deformed, husbandry is degraded with us, and the farmer leads the meanest of lives. He knows Nature but as a robber.[1]

—Henry David Thoreau, *Walden*

When I was a child, I spent many summer months on my uncle's farm in the Finger Lakes region of New York State. The house had no running water and smelled of the nineteenth century and had fascinating leftovers from its early days when it had orchards pruned and grafted almost into topiary, and outlying buildings for repairing rakes and cutters of various sorts, and a stately barn that smelled sweet with hay, oats, and wheat kernels.

I learned in those days when "I was happy as the grass was green," as Dylan Thomas puts it, that life on a farm is special, so naturally close to the growing and harvesting seasons and to the habits of animals, and open to the winds and rains and intense sunshine. In this passage Henry David Thoreau has a complaint that addresses one of his central themes and an issue close to my heart: the loss of the sacred in ordinary life.

No more processions. Thoreau may have been thinking of the Rogation Days in the Christian tradition. Begun in the early years of the sixth century, these liturgical festivals took place in late spring and included long formal walks through the fields as monks led the chanting of the litany of saints, a string of musical appeals to revered ones to bless the fields and crops and farmers. I remember being a young monk joining my community as we processed through the fields chanting the long litany and feeling in our bones the sacred nature of the fruitful earth.

But now the rituals are quiet. Nowadays you never see a line of monks walking seeded fields and chanting the names of saints. Nature has been desanctified. When an appreciation for the sacred in nature fails, we lose the very soul of our work and livelihood. It all becomes secular and soulless. Our work turns from priestly engagement with the earth to sheer labor in return for money.

Thoreau laments that in his day, as well, the sacred qualities of farming had been forgotten. Now food source and plots of earth are mere property and the farmer no longer an acolyte of the holy land but now a robber. What would he think of today's big business farms? Clearly, he felt strongly about the loss of the sacred to greed and exploitation. We have left behind, Thoreau says, the Roman goddess of agriculture Ceres, known to the Greeks as Demeter, a great mother goddess profoundly connected to her daughter Persephone, queen of the Underworld and goddess of spring. The ancient Greeks honored Demeter in their Eleusinian Mysteries, the main rituals in which the priestess displayed sheaves of grain pointing to the continuance of life, a way that farming cooperated with religion to give all who experienced the mysteries hope in the face of death.

Farmers know about life and death and are therefore acquainted with natural religion, if they are so inclined. It was said that my uncle, the farmer, could talk to animals. I saw them respond to the slightest twitch of his face or nod from his head. Like Thoreau, he did not like organized religion. Occasionally, the local Catholic priest would stop to see him and try to convince him to go to church, but my uncle would have none of it. I felt that his entire life was saturated with religion, even if the family worried about the state of his soul. Not all farmers are naturally religious, but some find direction in life from their intimacy with plants and animals.

Today America's most thoughtful writer on the farmer, Wendell Berry, in his essay "Economy and Pleasure," writes about work with a strong echo of Thoreau, whom he admires. He writes, "Ultimately, in the argument about work and how it should be done, one has only one's pleasure to offer. It is possible, as I have learned again and again, to be in one's place, in such company, wild or domestic, and with such pleasure, that one cannot think of another place that one would prefer to be—or of another place at all. One does not miss or regret the past, or fear or long for the future. Being there is simply all, and is enough."[2]

The farmer is more connected to his time, place, weather, and work than most other people are. As Wallace Stevens, said, "The poem is the cry of its occasion, Part of the res and not about it."[3] The farmer is more identified with their place than those who are not farmers. A farmer is part of the farm and not about it. You cannot abstract them from their field or even from their plants and animals, their barns and well-used kitchens. Thoreau would say, do not go into the forest with your books and thoughts. Just be there. Be the voice of the place.

We could all learn from the farmer to be more intimate with the world and allow it to shape life with its weather and play of light and darkness. We could all be an expression of the place where we live, but that would entail knowing the place well and firsthand. Identifying with the farmer could be the greatest lesson that Thoreau left us: the idea of being a natural person. Not just someone at home in nature but someone close to their own nature, an expression of the place and time in which you find yourself and a manifestation of the seeds of life that you have found in yourself and in the world, as it leads you toward your destiny.

Being a farmer is a sacred calling. Fortunate are those who can follow that calling and be shaped by the education in natural laws that farming entails. We might even evoke the great spirit of Demeter and Zeus in our gardening and in landscaping our homes and growing vegetables. A small effort in this direction has some potency, fortunately, because we cannot all be farmers. The important thing is to learn the ways of the earth and watch things grow and enjoy some intimacy with the chthonic gods of the ground.

Have we made a grievous mistake in creating huge capitalist, impersonal farms and watched the extinction of the family farm and its natural religion? When you consider that question, do you feel pressure from the thought that we need commercial farms to feed so many people? That could be a distraction from or a defense against keeping religion in our relation to both land and food. If, one day, we go back to inviting monks to process through our fields with their chants and blessings, we will know that the soulful farm has been restored.

14

WALDEN IN EDEN

Perhaps on that spring morning when Adam and Eve were driven out of Eden, Walden Pond was already in existence, and even then breaking up in a gentle spring rain, accompanied with mist and a southerly wind, and covered with myriads of ducks and geese, which had not heard of the fall, when still such sure lakes sufficed them. Even then it had commenced to rise and fall, and had clarified its waters and colored them of the hue they now wear, and obtained a patent of heaven to be the only Walden Pond in the world and distiller of celestial dews. Who knows in how many unremembered nations' literatures this has been the Castalian Fountain or what nymphs presided over it in the Golden Age? It is a gem of the first water which Concord wears in her coronet.[1]

—Henry David Thoreau, *Walden*

Henry David Thoreau left home to live apart and observe quietly and intensely as the elements, nature, neighbors, silence, and even beans gave him hints about his place in the world.

He discovered how to write about human values by living close to nature, seeing its ways through daily attention to animals, fish, and birds. Today, some people get a similar urge and go off by themselves to prepare for a new direction in life. I knew a man who followed his inner guide and went on retreat for a full year before beginning his life in medicine. My thirteen years of monastic study, from age thirteen to twenty-six, was a retreat of that kind for me, although I didn't understand it that way until later in life. Thoreau tells us why he chose a retreat at that moment: He wanted to live deliberately, not unconsciously. At the end he did not want to feel regret.

When Thoreau walked the short journey in miles but long in self-discovery, he was not traveling to the actual body of water and its forest but to the beginning of time, to Eden itself. He was starting over, accumulating what alchemists call *prima materia* (raw material), raw both in the trees and animals he met there and in the condition of his mind and heart.

Thoreau was good at boating down rivers, and his friend and guide Ralph Waldo Emerson had a special talent for working out important complex ideas by mastering words. Thoreau's words were also complex and strong and individual, but they were born from daily contact with farms and swamps and streams. Thoreau often contrasted his huckleberrying with the more financially secure and formal occupations of townies, preferring his vocation of berry picking over the more lucrative industry of the townspeople.

The friendship between Thoreau and Emerson was important for both, but it was not always harmonious. In spite of Emerson's significant gift of the land by Walden Pond, the two didn't live or work together at Walden, and yet Emerson's ideas, big heart, and excellence in expression lured Thoreau into a life of ideas and writing. They each had a creative genius, in the old sense of an indwelling presence, that drove them on in their lives. The friendship had its ups and downs, and Emerson's eulogy makes it clear that it was difficult at times. But neither man ever lost sight of it as a precious gift.

Emerson could see life's complexities with exceptional originality and then could light the torch in others who were inspired by his gift of language. He also had an elegant style that encouraged people to listen to him and want to learn from him. Emerson was a small-town squire, a public intellectual, and much lauded man. A neighbor of Emerson's said that the great man seemed to be ever walking on stilts.

Thoreau was a different kind of duck. At home in a small, homemade boat and observing plants and animals, he was Enkidu to Emerson's Gilgamesh. But to get a full picture of the experiment at Walden, you must take Emerson into account. Sometimes ideas and good sentences are more persuasive than personality.

While he was at Harvard, Thoreau read Emerson's grounding essay "Nature," in which the man who would be his friend and mentor wrote, "To speak truly, few adult persons can see nature. Most persons do not see the sun. . . . The lover of nature is he whose inward and outward senses are truly adjusted to each other."[2] Thoreau had two gifts that turned into a life work while he was living at Walden: skills for being in the natural world and a remarkable gift for writing. He approached nature outwardly and inwardly.

Thoreau lifts Walden Pond out of the literal context of an actual local lake, asking us to see its sacred and archetypal dimension. He places the pond in the mythic Garden of Eden, before time, in that region of prehistory the great religion scholar Mircea Eliade frequently referred to in Latin as *in illo tempore*, not in our time, but in *that* time, the time beyond time, the time of myth and mystery.

Thoreau describes Walden as "the distiller of celestial dews," not only the basin in which rain collects but the place where the mythic heavens shower their mysteries. When you read *Walden* or Thoreau's journals, you keep coming across passages where he mixes myth and natural phenomena. Thoreau verged toward being a scientific naturalist but never fully arrived there. The deep poet and natural theologian in him kept pulling him back to myth and the sacred.

Thoreau is a valuable guide for our time, when with our beloved secularism we struggle to make a future and a world. In the mid-nineteenth century and in his twenties, Thoreau was able to move toward a new kind of religion, a sacred sensibility focused on a mid-realm, neither literally religious nor dispassionately secular. The more you read his writings, the further you move into a realm of stunning mysteries and unexpected powers, a layer of experience where the secular and the sacred intermingle.

In Walden Pond, Thoreau's myth-tuned eyes perceived the Castalian Spring, in ancient Greece a source of water near the Oracle of Delphi. The pond did, in fact, serve as an oracle for Thoreau, who wrote, "A lake is the landscape's most beautiful and expressive feature. It is earth's eye; looking into which the beholder measures the depth of his own nature."[3]

Today we lack the wisdom to consult oracles in nature seriously. We have lost the spiritual and imaginative skills needed to hear the invisible voices that offer direction. We think we are superior to the ancients, but our dominant philosophy is so factual and literal that we have little access to the natural spirits that could guide and sustain us. We are too far removed from the realm of dream, which could temper our materialism and reveal a deeper way. Why not look at a local body of water and imagine that it was there at the beginning of creation, in the mythic Garden of Eden.

While it is true in general, it is especially important in Thoreau's mind that when imagination is in play, the spiritual and the sacred can thrive. One serves the other. To look at Walden Pond and see Eden is the measure of a profoundly awakened person, someone who appreciates William Blake's famous verse: "May God us keep us from Single vision & Newton's sleep." The Newtonian eye looks and sees a small lake in a landscape of other ponds. But someone wakened in the way of Blake and Thoreau sees Eden and Delphi brought to life in those local waters.

Modern life does not afford us two kinds of time: This time that we measure with clocks and calendars and that time that touches on the timeless. For Thoreau, Walden came from the time and space of the gods, so leaving his home to live by the pond was to move closer to the deepest mysteries of life. Today many people cling desperately to moralistic and literalistic religion but lack the capacity to find Eden in their local world.

The difference here lies in the basic imaginative lens we use to see. For Thoreau, neither the lens of science nor of institutional religion nor of common sense offer a landscape that he wanted to inhabit. At Walden, he cultivated an alternate reality. He not only escaped the Newtonian culture of money and industry, he rediscovered the enchanted realm of myth and sacredness.

There is no reason why we could not do the same: Abandon our culture of greed and narrow vision and rediscover, as the natural man Henry David Thoreau did, a refuge of myth and profound meaning, where values are deep and connections with nature far-reaching and, in the best sense, mystical.

15

BE COLD AND HUNGRY

Take long walks in stormy weather or through deep snows in the fields and woods, if you would keep your spirits up. Deal with brute nature. Be cold and hungry and weary.[1]

—Henry David Thoreau, journal entry, December 25, 1856

How do you keep your spirits up? Do you eat a good dinner, go for a stroll, watch a movie? Henry David Thoreau has a different idea. Take a long walk in stormy weather. Trudge through deep snow. Be cold and hungry and weary.

Thoreau is often a contrarian, someone who does the opposite of what seems right or convenient. He defines himself as a nonconformer. He distances himself from normal social reality. He would keep his spirits up by walking in stormy weather.

Modern life is one massive attempt to avoid the storms and deep snows of life. We appreciate conveniences and even have stores named for that purpose. Whenever possible we want to take the easy route and live always in fair weather. In another journal entry, Thoreau says that we can often enjoy the best landscape in the worst weather. As many painters and photographers would attest, the beauty of a place really shines in stormy conditions. How many movie scenes play out against the sound of thunder and the flash of lightning? Mary Shelley was inspired to write *Frankenstein* during a remarkable storm. A friend of mine from England, Andrew Machon, travels intrepidly to the snowy Arctic Circle to photograph the aurora borealis.

I have often noted that during my practice of psychotherapy a client might phone me late at night asking for an appointment at the next possible time. On the other hand, no one ever called late to say that things were going well and they would like an appointment tomorrow. The urgency, the emotional storm encouraged them to focus on their well-being and attend to their souls. It is an obvious but essential lesson: urgency and emotional pressure, storm clouds, lead directly to therapy. James Hillman often said similarly that depression takes us to a gray environment where you can see and feel important things not accessible anywhere else.

Picture Thoreau, the man, happier on a river with a few fruits and vegetables stored away on his small, homemade boat than comfortable in a tavern or a fine home. These preferences reveal the nature of the man, how he lives and thinks and why he might be someone worth listening to. Like Thoreau, we could choose not to live the easy life, but rather find beauty in the challenge. We might even seek out the storm.

Thoreau's retreat to Walden Pond was not just a quest for solitude, but an attempt to live closer to the elements, the seasons of beans, and the ways of muskrats and sunfish. He learned that these stubborn citizens of outdoors confronted him with their needs and expectations. Even on retreat in solitude, he could not live any way he liked. By responding to nature's demands, Thoreau found that his own most intimate self was revealed. He found a power for self-unfolding that was not his ego.

Thoreau lived in two realms, and he approached both with ardor: the messy ways of an explorer and the confronting ways of the writer. One of the great mysteries of his life, an element that we would do well to emulate, is the process of transmuting encounters with nature into art, effectively putting one word after another, if only in conversation.

It is a mistake to think of Thoreau only as the first environmentalist or the intrepid explorer. He gave much of his life to study, reading, and writing. At first, he thought he would be a poet, as Ralph Waldo Emerson encouraged him, but then he discovered painfully that he did not have the gifts of a real poet. Instead, he developed his own prose style, with its subtle allusions, wry hyperbole, and vivid landscaping.

When you read Thoreau, you can see that even as a writer he chose to take walks on stormy days and nights. No eternal sunshine for him. He worked hard at mining language for beauty and insight. He avoided cliché and well-worn truisms, dangers in his subject matter. He also took pains to develop a style, and even a character. In *Walden*, especially, he is not so much the subject of the writing but the main character in a collection of tales.

Thoreau was willing to walk into the fray, as when he famously spent a night in jail for not paying a tax. He and his family also stepped into a storm when they participated fully in the Underground Railroad, keeping freedom seekers in their home. Thoreau was vocal about his support for the emancipationist John Brown, and he took risks escorting enslaved people to Canada.

To keep your spirits up, deal with brute nature, Thoreau says. I take this philosophy to mean that you should face the confronting issues in your life, whether on a personal level or in society. Take on a challenge rather than wait for it to be resolved by others. Do nothing or simply wait only if you want to be unhappy.

The decision to be strong rather than passive can help prevent any masochistic acceptance of abuse. You can trace back certain strains of sadness to a moment when you allowed someone or something to take away your power and agency. It knocks the wind, the life spirit, out of you, and you feel defeated. Thoreau was able to maintain his personal power in day-to-day situations that were not heroic or massive in scope. He simply used eccentricity and chronic contrariness to maintain his individual presence in what he perceived as a crowd of soul-snatchers.

Emerson said in his eulogy that Thoreau wasn't an easy man to be close to. "There was somewhat military in his nature not to be subdued, always manly and able, but rarely tender, as if he did not feel himself except in opposition. He wanted a fallacy to expose, a blunder to pillory, I may say required a little sense of victory, a roll of the drum, to call his powers into full exercise. It cost him nothing to say No; indeed, he found it much easier than to say Yes."[2]

For myself, I was born a quiet person; at times, you could say, passive. I would like a dose of Thoreau's roll of the drum in me, but I expect to remain peaceable rather than militant. You don't have to be like Thoreau, either, but you can learn from him. Understand that he was able to adopt a persona that was in tune with his ideas and models a way that is narrow and easily abused. Still, "walk into a storm" might be a better piece of advice than stand around and hope for good weather.

16

THE COLD BLOOD OF THE GODS

I am glad to hear that you were there too. There are many more such voyages, and longer ones, to be made on that river, for it is the water of life. The Ganges is nothing to it. Observe its reflections,—no idea but is familiar to it. That river, though to dull eyes it seems terrestrial wholly, flows through Elysium. What powers bathe in it invisible to villagers! Talk of its shallowness,—that hay-carts can be driven through it at midsummer: its depth passeth my understanding. If, forgetting the allurements of the world, I could drink deeply enough of it; if cast adrift from the shore, I could with complete integrity float on it, I should never be seen on the mill-dam again. If there is any depth in me, there is a corresponding depth in it. It is the cold blood of the gods. I paddle and bathe in their artery.[1]

—Henry David Thoreau to Harrison
Gray Otis Blake, December 9, 1855

Henry David Thoreau is an outstanding human being for being so sensitive to nature, for treating animals as his cousins, and for keeping the forest as a park and the swamp close to the town and city. These are accomplishments that could help us live more intimately on our planet. But perhaps more important is his lesson here about seeing. The great Indigenous leader Black Elk taught us to see "in a sacred manner" and in that way behold the secrets of life and how to live. Thoreau's greater contribution to humanity is to teach how to get beyond looking at life through "dull eyes" that cannot see Elysium or Eden from a simple stream or flowing river. What to call this different kind of seeing? Mythic, enchanted, magical, archetypal, sacred?

We have extraordinary tools and instruments, such as telescopes and microscopes, to help us *look at* the natural world, but Thoreau offers clues for *seeing* the world as it relates to us. The distinction between looking and seeing is crucial. A telescope is mainly for looking, while a hike up a mountain or a paddle down a stream is for seeing, because the place and our way of being in it transform and enchant, and we begin to see what is invisible to "wholly terrestrial" eyes, eyes focused only to see the literal and the factual. For Thoreau, the rivers and the pond where he lived, offering enchantment and magic, were portals to myth.

In the seventeenth century an unusual alchemist and cosmic philosopher, Robert Fludd, published his major work on the great cosmos of the world and the corresponding microcosm of the human being. One of his many inventive images depicts a man looking out at the world from the third eye that is up front in his skull. Other images in that illustration depict seven layers of reality. Thoreau, too, goes out into the woods with his third eye and his several levels of vision and his *oculus imaginationis* (eye of imagination), and sees more than an ordinary person ever has.

"That river, though to dull eyes it seems terrestrial wholly, flows through Elysium," Thoreau writes to his friend Harrison Gray Otis

Blake. Dull eyes are not up in the skull, not eyes of imagination. They do not see the river flowing through Elysium, which traditionally is a place of pleasure and reward in the afterlife, a kind of paradise. Thoreau had such good intracranial eyesight that he could see Eden and the Ganges, as well. He understood that sacred places on Earth, like the Ganges and the Euphrates Rivers, are holy, set apart, in a special realm of imagination. They are not limited to a factual place but are omnipresent. They are essential to everyone on the planet and can be conjured in local rivers and forests. All that is required is the eye that sees through the eggshell surface of reality.

If you really want to adopt Thoreau's Walden worldview, you should go out into the natural world often, but always with eyes transformed by some poetic powder that empowers you to see the gods and their terrain. You see the local river but also spot the mythology that streams beneath and within the streaming.

The actual river Thoreau is talking about is the Assabet, which flows southwest of Concord and branches into the Concord River in the town of Concord. It is a small, shallow river, but a beautiful one in which several kinds of fish could be seen in Thoreau's day. In the letter quoted, he describes a trip he made to collect firewood in his small boat. He encourages his Worcester friend, Otis Blake, to go boating on that river, because it is the "water of life," *aqua vitae*. In the Gospel story of Jesus and the woman at the well, the two discuss this special water, not H_2O, but the water of life that sprouts a spiritualizing imagination and the capacity to see myth levitating somewhere between the surface of the stream and the bedrock.

On any river or lake you and I could find ourselves in *aqua vitae*, but we would need that special eye that sees beyond the literal. Thoreau had it, and for him it made all the difference. It allowed him to be out in nature and glimpse there the sacred landscape he needed for a meaningful life. At the outset of his Walden experiment he said he went out "to meet the facts of life—the vital facts, which are the phenomena or actuality the gods meant to show us, face to face."[2]

We moderns for the most part imagine divinity as a being somewhere among the clouds, engineering, or even puppeteering, life on earth. The theology of many adults has not penetrated the literal, and in these special matters they still think factually rather than spiritually. But Thoreau had a good education in the classics, where he would find a path toward theological sophistication. He knew that divinity is less humanlike and less physical than the modern untutored eye sees it, and therefore he could speak directly of divinity in the natural realm. The infinite became palpable in the woods or on the river, and in a reflective float down the winding and ever-charming Assabet he could detect the nature spirits that nourish the soul.

The Assabet River is shallow enough to drive a hay cart through it in summer, and yet to Thoreau this river has impressive depth. If you have the eye of imagination, a beautiful, shallow river will have depth of meaning for you. A shallow anything can have immense depth and will nourish you in spite of its actual dimensions. This is just one of Thoreau's general rules of perception: Don't be misled by anything measured in inches. The depth of a river is not measured by its dimensions but by its beauty and character. Its depth is not measurable but qualitative.

See your neighboring rivers as the arteries of the gods. Do not live at a superficial level that is blind to such a discovery. Put on the eyeglasses of myth and penetrate beyond the literal to appreciate a dimension that will truly speak to your deepest self. This exhortation is similar to William Blake's dictum: "If the doors of perception were cleansed every thing would appear to man as it is, Infinite. For man has closed himself up, till he sees all things thro' narrow chinks of his cavern."[3]

17

CLODHOPPER THAT I AM

You may rely on it that you have the best of me in my books, and that I am not worth seeing personally—the stuttering . . . blundering, clod-hopper that I am.

I should be surprised and alarmed if there were any great call for me. I confess that I am considerably alarmed even when I hear that an individual wishes to meet me, for my experience teaches me that we shall thus only be made certain of a mutual strangeness which otherwise we might never have been aware of.

—Henry David Thoreau to Calvin Harlow Greene, February 10, 1856

As for compliments,—even the stars praise me, and I praise them.—They & I sometimes belong to a mutual admiration society.[1]

—Henry David Thoreau to Harrison Gray Otis Blake, March 13, 1856

Many in Henry David Thoreau's circle agreed with him that he was a clodhopper. In his eulogy, Ralph Waldo Emerson said: "No college ever offered him a diploma, or a professor's chair; no academy made him its corresponding secretary, its discoverer, or even its member. Perhaps these learned bodies feared the satire of his presence . . . He grew to be revered and admired by his townsmen, who had at first known him only as an oddity."

"The satire of his presence." A remarkable description of a man whose writing is so artfully shaped and perfected. But Thoreau knew that he was blundering and stuttering. Perhaps Emerson means that if Thoreau were to become a member of an honored society, that group might be embarrassed by him. He would not fit into any self-respecting organization because he would want to go his own way, which, by his own account, was rough and contrary. He would turn out to be a spoof of the very society of which he was a member. He was always and essentially a clodhopper, forever leaping over clods of mud, and truth be told, enjoying his rustic setting far more than polite town society.

His mere presence could force some people to acknowledge their fussiness and in that way, too, offer satire. But what made Thoreau's clodhopper quality special was that he was knowledgeable about many things, and, as Emerson says, would be sought after for his expertise in many areas. He was not the full-blown clodhopper he imagined himself to be. He was more like the author of *Walden*, who could write beautifully in a country sort of way, and then be awkward at a party. He was full of contradictions, and so he didn't think it was worth anyone's effort to meet him in person. In contrast, you would never expect to hear such a thing from Emerson.

Throughout Thoreau's writing you find him dismissing learned societies and high culture. He especially picked on classical music performed in polite society, saying he would rather hear the music of crickets than attend an opera in the city. A lover of classical music myself, I bristle at Thoreau's frequent takedown of it. High culture can certainly become overly formal and fastidious, and Thoreau did not hesitate to complain of it. As I see it, he had a talent for an earthy, animal-like way of life, and that lifestyle might have inclined him against the formalities of society. His guiding spirit was Pan, the wild, high-stepping god of nature, rather than Apollo with his stately lyre.

The poet Wendell Berry has often been associated with Thoreau. He writes: "As Thoreau so well knew, and so painstakingly tried to show us, what a man most needs is not a knowledge of how to get more, but a knowledge of the most he can do without, and of how to get along without it."[2]

In this philosophy of appreciating what you do not have Thoreau is again a clodhopper. Most people measure their happiness and success in life by what they have. Meanwhile, Thoreau is out in the field, happy as can be, jumping over clumps of earth that he does not own, feeling wealthy because of the mud on his shoes.

Thoreau's nonconformity may be understood under the umbrella of transcendentalism and its creed of self-reliance. In the essay of that name, Emerson wrote: "Whoso would be a man, must be a nonconformist." When he realized that he could not be a minister in a liberal church in Boston, he had to face his own "aboriginal self" (his phrase), the identity given to him before his birth, his destiny. Emerson didn't have the clodhopper calling of Thoreau, but he was eccentric in his own way.

As I have written and lectured about soul over thirty years, I have often advocated eccentricity, although it is not obvious in my own presence. In fact, my eccentricity is to be normal and low-key. One of my clients, who dresses and lives like a self-expressive artist, once asked me with worry in his voice, "If I become a therapist, do I have to wear a white shirt and blue sweater, like you do?" In other words, do I have to be so uninteresting?

Once, I gave a lecture at a large university, and true to my own high estimation of higher learning, I wore a suit and tie. This was some years ago when it was still fashionable to dress up for such occasions. After the talk, a young man came up to me and said, "I traveled far to come hear you speak. I have been impressed with the originality of your ideas. But here I see a most conventional man, dressed in a suit with neat hair and polite manners. I'm disappointed, to say the least. I expected you, of all people, to show us how to be unique and expressive." I told the man I was sorry to disappoint him, but this is who I am. I am ordinary. My goal is to be nonconformist to nonconformity. I am a clodhopper in my own way and sometimes feel like a misfit in my unremarkable normality.

When we say the soul is timeless, you may consider that it stands outside of time and is anachronistic. Or, your soul may not be adapted to society, and so you appear to others as an outsider. I recommend being like Thoreau and admitting unabashedly to the clodhopper in you. You don't demean yourself. You just present yourself as who you are and take a little pleasure in not meeting expectations. I suspect that some clodhoppers are afraid of normality and therefore retreat into their oddness. They could use my strategy and treat normality as outlandish.

To my readers I can use Thoreau's very words: "You may rely on it that you have the best of me in my books, and that I am not worth seeing personally—the stuttering, blundering, clod-hopper that I am." I do not stutter, but I do blunder, and I am often shy, reticent, and awkward. People do say that I walk my talk, and that impresses them, but for myself I would rather meet your acquaintance in the pages of one of my books. There, the clodhopper seems to be largely closeted.

I also recommend that you cultivate for yourself an "inner clodhopper." In whatever ways you falter or appear uncouth or out of place, your creativity lies in being at home. At its root, *uncouth* means unknown, not recognized, or not yet seen. It is not so bad. People have not yet seen the character you are, and so your inferior self offers you a degree of originality.

Thoreau's clodhopping turned into a writing style that has charmed and educated people for almost two hundred years. It is there in the noblest of his sentences and has become identified with his appealing voice. Take the clodhopper out of Thoreau and the brilliant *Walden* might disappear from our libraries.

18

THE FERN SCRIPTURES

If you would make acquaintance with the ferns you must forget your botany. You must get rid of what is commonly called knowledge of them. You must be aware that nothing is what you have taken it to be. In what book is this world and its beauty described? . . . if it is required that you be affected by ferns, that they amount to anything, signify anything to you, that they be another sacred scripture and revelation to you, helping to redeem your life, this end is not so surely accomplished. . . . I do not know how to distinguish between waking life and a dream. Are we not always living the life we imagine we are? . . . Each green tuft of ferns is a grove where some nobility dwells and walks—the concentrated greenness of the swamp.[1]

—Henry David Thoreau, journal entries,
October 4, 1859, and November 12, 1859

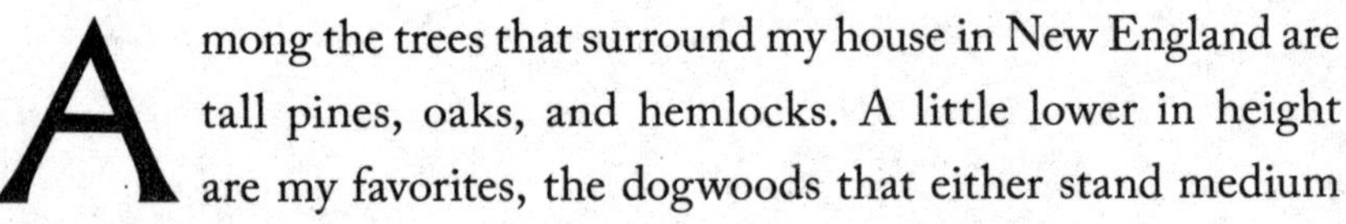

Among the trees that surround my house in New England are tall pines, oaks, and hemlocks. A little lower in height are my favorites, the dogwoods that either stand medium high or bend over to reach the sunlight pouring through the rhododendrons. Far lower and spreading over all the land around are the green ferns that seem magical, being so delicate and different in shape from all the rest. These ferns have the distinction of having brought their green coverage to Earth's forests 160 million years ago. They may be frail, but they are long-lived.

Henry David Thoreau describes the ferns as sacred scripture, revealing essential secrets and truths for our redemption. They serve the forest as angels serve the heavens—protective, beautiful, and, above all, green. One Latin name for the fern is pteridophyte, *pteri* meaning "feather." Ferns are wings on the soil, introducing a green ethereality like the blue angels Thoreau glimpsed on Walden Pond. They sanctify a place. In their simplicity they exaggerate the purpose of plants to nurture, grow, and multiply.

In theology, scripture is not just any writing, but a message written by the hand of God, a message from on high. Thoreau would not push that language far, but he would say that ferns offer teachings that come from divinity itself, and their message is a saving one. With their very greenness they could save us from being caught in the brown-dry wasteland of culture. They urge us to recover our own plant nature and come back to life.

The expressive power of the fern lies primarily in color, the special green of the plant that helps make a forest or a garden a lush display of what Hildegard of Bingen called *viriditas*, the green essence, the vital power of plant existence. To focus on the particular green of nature is to recover a sense of belonging and beginning. You can uncover your own green life, but to do so, you must see the ferns and not just look at them.

Dylan Thomas's inspired, bouncy poem "Fern Hill" associates the color green with youth and vitality. Viriditas is an alternative to and a tonic for the vacancy that is life without deep awareness and soul.

Thomas describes himself in the poem as "happy as the grass was green." Viriditas, revealed so richly in the common fern, brings happiness as well as growth and youth.

In the thirteenth century, the theologian Thomas Aquinas wrote philosophically about a plant or vegetative soul. All animate beings have such a soul, he says, which allows for three necessary conditions: nutrition, growth, and generation. This means, as I read it, that you and I have a plant soul. Just as we say that we are animal in nature, so we are all, at one level, plants. We sometimes say that we are human animals, but we are also human plants. Specifically, we have a fern nature, a sort of Buddha nature of the forest, the power to nurture yourself, grow, and generate. We are fern green, accessible to viriditas, continually revitalized by the green principle.

More precisely, we may all also have a fern soul. When you are in the presence of a fern, you are seeing that generally hidden aspect of yourself that is of the plant family. You are greeting your cousin, as Thoreau might put it. You share a life with that plant, so it is no wonder that you enjoy living with it and having it in and around your home.

Ferns signify many things to different people. To one person they may be something natural in an artificial environment. To another they are a common and unimportant plant, used for easy decoration. Others, of course, love this plant, and in all parts of the world it has been a token of bounty and good luck. Thoreau places ferns in the sphere of natural religion. A fern is ordinary beyond explaining, and yet it may save you from a worthless life. It redeems you and reveals your deep, green essence.

To redeem means to pay your debt and recover your worthiness. In Christian theology it refers to Jesus dying torturously to pay the price for the sins of humankind. But how does a fern save you? For one, it reveals who and what you are. You are a gossamer plant, tenuous and delicate. If you know this secret of human mythic biology, you can focus some of your self-care, even self-culture, on that dimension of the self.

A fern lives its precarious life so that we humans can have pleasure. It saves us from ugliness and a world without nature's backdrop. The unimportance of ferns, their lowliness, especially, saves us in ordinary circumstances, where we can't afford a flashier plant. In their low place in the world of plant hierarchy, they pay a hefty price for giving us a mere sample of beauty. They don't grow from seed, they don't flower, and they get sick easily from a bad balance of moisture and sun. They are delicate and frail in some ways, strong in others.

Ferns do not dominate like a sunflower, but cower low to the ground, almost unseen in their shyness. Thoreau frequently appealed to the common man, the ordinary person, the unexceptional being who would be closer to the deep pulse of things and bring more important contributions to the world. He appreciated the ferns among humans.

Ferns are a revelation of nature's patience. Ferns don't need innovation or any change in style. They reveal a quiet sameness that is a characteristic of timeless being. In this way they embody the infinite, the divinity in nature that Thoreau begged us to take into account. They could remind us of the eternal in us, that which doesn't change or depend on development. We might learn from ferns to celebrate the changeless in human life, instead of the new inventions and styles that we seem to prefer. If we remained in touch with the eternal, green dimension of our soul, we might find the peace that the fern has enjoyed for millions of years. We might rest easy in the quiet nooks of the forest and enjoy our green lowliness and simplicity.

19

THE APPLE TREE BUILDING

Flint's Pond! Such is the poverty of our nomenclature. What right had the unclean and stupid farmer, whose farm abutted on this sky water, whose shores he has ruthlessly laid bare, to give his name to it? Some skin-flint, who loved better the reflecting surface of a dollar, or a bright cent, in which he could see his own brazen face; who regarded even the wild ducks which settled in it as trespassers; his fingers grown into crooked and horny talons from the long habit of grasping harpy-like,—so it is not named for me. I go not there to see him nor to hear of him; who never saw it, who never bathed in it, who never loved it, who never protected it, who never spoke a good word for it, nor thanked God that he had made it. Rather, let it be named from the fishes that swim in it, the wild fowl or quadrupeds which frequent it, the wild flowers which grow by its shores, or some wild man or child the thread of whose history is interwoven with its own.[1]

—Henry David Thoreau, *Walden*

Once, I was staying at a hotel in downtown Chicago. One morning I walked out of the hotel onto a busy street and looked up to check the weather. The first thing I saw was a building across the narrow, noisy street with a familiar name in huge brassy letters. It was the name of a popular politician at the time. Immediately I felt uneasy. Why should I be out in a favorite city of mine looking at morning clouds, hoping to behold the spirit of the place, and instead find a man's name in my face, bold and insistent, blotting out the city and the sky? I felt the slap of egotism, an expression of superiority that makes you feel diminished and stands between you and life.

I have had similar feelings at college campuses, where bright new buildings often carry the names of donors and benefactors. I am truly grateful for people who support education, but does that mean they should have their names on buildings and parks? Does naming have a deeper function than to tout financial largess?

I feel the way Henry David Thoreau does, who in this passage seems upset about the custom of naming ponds and woods and other natural areas for donors and owners. He says, find someone who loved the place or lived there and linked their life and identity to it. Better to name it after a fish, or a flower, or even an insect. The Rose Building, or Barracuda Plaza, or even Praying Mantis Park would be an improvement over John Smith Woods. The name of a place steers our imaginations and emotions in a certain direction. Wouldn't it be better to be reminded of a natural mystery rather than a person's bank account?

Naming buildings and other public places after wealthy benefactors may suggest excessive capitalism, honoring an individual whose value is measured mainly by financial success, stroking an ego to receive a gift, and pressure to grant the donor further influence or control. These are my own thoughts, but today serious work is being done on the ethics of fundraising, which includes examining the process of naming buildings and places.

We find in Thoreau that this question, not much discussed in public, is a serious one that he felt strongly about. One reason would be that the focus on financial wealth associated with naming obscures higher values such as nature, art, and humanity. If you walk around a college campus and see one park or building after another named for wealth and power, your experience of that place will be colored by these honorifics in a certain direction. It is a matter of ecology.

Buildings are like persons. They stand in our midst and relate to us, whether we want them to or not. They affect us with their strong presence, and they can have a wide variety of character. They are part of the commons, which was so dear to Thoreau and could be for us. Donors' names can take away from the aura of commons. Put up a building in a neighborhood, and you make a longstanding and prominent change. Everyone must adapt to it and will have feelings and ideas about it. Maybe we should collectively name our buildings and parks. Maybe they should serve community rather than personality.

Thoreau would rather honor the animal and plant life of a place than respond to one person's need for recognition. He liked to name places and would sometimes use a name of his choosing for a place, even if the place already had a name. He would say, "This is what I call Otter Bay."[2] When I saw the politician's self-promoting building in Chicago, instead of being annoyed, I could have renamed it. Passing Cloud would have worked well for me.

For all his complaints about Farmer Flint, Thoreau named some places after farmers and other citizens of Concord. Flint must have so annoyed Thoreau that he would not use the name Flint as a point of honor. We, too, might want to name places for people who are of special remembrance, like John Muir, Martin Luther King Jr., Toni Morrison, or Georgia O'Keeffe. Thoreau's outrage applies to the person who has contributed money without having any intimacy with the place.

Just as your name is full of meaning and identity, a building or a pond's name affects the soul of the place. It is not a label—it is an evocation of values and history. The name directs us how to think of the place and relate to it. It helps us befriend the building, an object that needs friends.

Names, especially when they are prominently attached to a building, are like statues of the genius loci, the resident spirit of a place, which in Roman times might be a roughly carved stone. The stone gives body to the spirit of the place and helps people sense its presence. Do we want the spirit of personal wealth or, like Thoreau, do we want to acknowledge an animal or plant?

Our world shrinks when we replace a spirit of nature with personal ambition and control. Maybe spending time in the forest, as Thoreau did, might help us get our values straight and name our buildings and places accordingly.

Liverpool, England, takes its name from Old English words for "dark water." Dublin, Ireland, has its name from the Irish words for "dark pool." Liverpool is full of images of the liver bird, actually a cormorant, which is well-known in the area. Florence is from "flower," and Hong Kong means "fragrant harbor." Thoreau took pride in the name of his beloved town Concord, a variant of "peace."

Naming is an aspect of self-culture, which the transcendentalists championed and that Ellery Channing defined, writing, "Like a plant or animal, the nobler qualities of any individual can also grow, and if that individual does what he can to unfold all his powers and capacities, especially his nobler ones, he practices self-culture."[3] Naming is at attempt to grow culture and could be a process of ennobling.

When we name a thing, we could be close to our better selves and able to employ all our powers. Naming is a kind of baptism, incorporating the building into the community. Certainly, sometimes we name a park or a building after a person who gave their life for the community, to be reminded of these values. There is nothing wrong with money, but in certain contexts it may not express the values a community cherishes or grows on. If I worked on a college campus or in a business park, I would be happy to have my office in Butterfly Plaza or Red Ant Towers.

20
THE EYELIDS OF THE DAY

All transcendent goodness is one, though appreciated in different ways, or by different senses. In beauty we see it, in music we hear it, in fragrance we scent it. In the palatable the pure palate tastes it and in rare health the whole body feels it. The variety is in the surface or manifestation; but the radical identity we fail to express. The lover sees in the glance of his beloved the same beauty that in the sunset paints the western skies. It is the same daimon, here lurking under a human eyelid and there under the closing eyelids of the day. Here, in small compass, is the ancient and natural beauty of evening and morning. What loving astronomer has ever fathomed the ethereal depths of the eye?[1]

—Henry David Thoreau to Harrison Gray
Otis Blake, September 23, 1852

In this inspired passage, Henry David Thoreau is the Platonist or Neoplatonist, even the depth psychologist who directs his attention to the eternal powers that generate life and wisdom in us, the archetypal psychologist (psyche-logos) who values psyche or soul and who embodies logos in a profound pursuit of poetic and mystical gnosis. He looks far more deeply than the average genius into layers of experience that lie beneath sense impressions or typical analyses or standard ideas, far more deeply than the usual modernist who treats everything on the surface and fails to penetrate to the mysterious, the truly philosophical, and the genuinely religious. Here, speaking of the correspondences between human love and natural phenomena, Thoreau takes on the role of shaman, one who exists in and traverses several layers of experience and can move between worlds and see with an eye that is not locked in facts and measurements.

A passage like this moves me to venture a portrait of Thoreau that goes beyond nature as a fact, so that he is not a naturalist, essentially, but a mystic philosopher in search of a meaningful, layered world. He is a human being in that world animated by this vision, and an individual who yearns to uncover his own place in life and his own unique path. Nature is the instrument of his vision, not the object. The world in which he lives—the town of Concord and the trees and plants and animals encircling his home on Walden Pond—feed his mysticism, which is the true nature of his labor. It is not unusual in history for a mystic to be surrounded by nature—St. Francis of Assisi and Hildegard of Bingen, to name two.

We have many modes of sensing the first layer of reality. We look and listen and feel and see. In the arts we start with the senses and immediately find ourselves in a realm of mysteries. In this way art and the spiritual are indescribably close, as for Thoreau, nature and natural religion go hand in hand.

The deepest layer we cannot put into words or maybe even thought. Here we get hints of the archetypal, the eternal mass within the ordinary world of time. It is beyond words. We wander our way around it to arrive at hints and suggestions of what it is. In an ancient manner, the sentiment is found in such mystical philosophers as Plotinus, Marsilio Ficino, Robert Fludd, and even in Thoreau's friend Margaret Fuller. The woman who could, and perhaps should have been, his friend, the unknown neighbor Emily Dickinson, also understood that the love that keeps the planets in motion and the seasons on schedule and trees in community is the same love that draws one person into love with another. "It is the same daimon, here lurking under a human eyelid and there under the closing eyelids of the day." It could not be said better.

Here we can add Thoreau to a long list of mystical magicians, philosophers, and depth psychologists who conceive of human life as daimonic. Homer, Herakleitos, Socrates, Jesus, Marsilio Ficino, Nicholas of Cusa, William Butler Yeats, Rollo May, Carl Jung, James Hillman, and even in their own language Lao Tzu and Zhuang Zhou. They all based their reflections concerning the source of human awareness and character on the notion of daimon, a mysterious other, which originally was a nameless spirit that guides and empowers the human being. We do not create our own identities but are made by the forces in life that inspire us and with which we sometimes struggle.

The beauty of a lover and the beauty of a sunset are the same. Thoreau refers to this beauty as a daimon. What is glanced and appreciated as beauty is the daimon, the pulse of life in the shape of something beautiful, a powerful force that can make life worthwhile and can inspire rapture. Sometimes the daimon is felt inwardly as an urge or an inhibition, but it could appear as the natural potency in the sun or a body of water.

You can live your life by means of these daimonic messages. Sometimes the daimon is out in the world, as a person who has a powerful impact on your life, as an idea or approach that makes everything tolerably clear, or as a piece of art that focuses all your experiences and understandings. For me, Johann Sebastian Bach's Keyboard

Concerto in F Minor has such a daimonic force, but so do Ludwig van Beethoven's Seventh Symphony, Igor Stravinsky's *The Firebird*, and Willie Nelson's version of "Blue Skies."

Thoreau glimpsed the daimonic in the natural world around him, in small things like crickets and frogs, and in big things like local mountains that pointed to the meaning of his life. Thoreau lived daimonically and therefore not so humanly, except as the daimonic can give your humanity thrust and taste. But there is something frightening in a daimonic presence. You don't treat it like a pet kitten, even if it is as alien to humans as an animal. You respect its virulence and understand that as potentially explosive it is, so much a part of nature and a grace to humans.

In the many magical paintings of Annunciation in art history, you are reminded of the story in Luke 1:35 in which an angel appears to the Virgin Mary and says:

> A holy spirit will come over you and
> the power of the highest will envelop you in shadow
> and the holy being to be born
> will be called a son of God.

The "holy spirit" is a daimon, one that in this story brings new, cosmic life to the world in the form of a small child. Any artist, any human being, can be visited by an angelic being and be advised that the daimon is near and life will change. I was once visited by a powerful daimon that instructed me to be a monk. I couldn't have refused it if I wanted to. That visitor infused my entire life and introduced me to my future. There have been other visitations, as well.

Even though the daimon of Eros, which Socrates spoke of, brings us deeper into life, time and again, it is a humanizing power. Great nature and human experience share the same guidance. "The lover sees in the glance of his beloved the same beauty that in the sunset paints the western skies."

In all of Thoreau's examinations of nature he is also always looking for signs of the divine or the daimonic, always in search of meaning for human beings and for his own existence. The world and I share more than ever appears. By looking deep into the forest and far into the stars of night I discover myself and cherish that vision the way I cherish life with my life partner. And when I behold and love the eyelids of my companion, I am preparing to take note of the eyelids of the universe revealed from the perspective of my planet.

21

THE HOARY BLOOM

I see in the path some rank thimble-berry shoots covered with that peculiar hoary bloom very thickly. It is only rubbed off in a few places down to the purple skin, by some passing hunter perchance. It is a very singular and delicate outer coat, surely, for a plant to wear. I find that I can write my name in it with a pointed stick very distinctly, each stroke, however fine, going down to the purple. It is a new kind of enamelled card.

What is this bloom, and what purpose does it serve? Is there anything analogous in animated nature? It is the coup de grace, the last touch and perfection of any work, a thin elysian veil cast over it, through which it may be viewed. It is breathed on by the artist, and thereafter his work is not to be touched without injury. It is the evidence of a ripe and completed work, on which the unexhausted artist has breathed out of his superfluous genius, and his work looks through it as a veil.

If it is a poem, it must be invested with a similar bloom by the imagination of the reader. It is the subsidence of superfluous

> *ripeness. Like a fruit preserved in its own sugar. It is the handle by which the imagination grasps it.*[1]
>
> —Henry David Thoreau, journal entry, November 4, 1857

Many plants, like blueberries, have a frosty whitish coat over the blue skin called a bloom. In furniture it is a waxy coating dabbed on an object or enamel paint that dries to a hard, shiny finish. As is his custom, Henry David Thoreau compares this bloom to the polish one can detect on an excellent work of art, not a literal final coat but a sheen of finish and possibly perfection, as when you finish reading a poem and declare it wondrous. The spirit of the thing remains as an afterglow or a blush on fine wine. You sense this in people, too, grasping that they have lived their lives generously and courageously and then leave with a wondrous afterpresence.

At the end of James Hillman's book on aging, *The Force of Character*, there is a chapter titled "Finish." He writes, "'Finished' also means finely wrought, highly polished, like the sheen on worn, well-waxed wood. What is left after leaving is the actual state of character, the way the years have put a finish on it and not merely to it."[2]

But finishes can happen throughout life, especially in the work we do and the things we create. I can tell when a book is done, as Hillman says, not when it is finished but when it has a finish, something like the blue haze on evening mountains or the grayish blush on ripe blueberries. In creative activity, finish is more subtle. You see the completed thing—say, a painting—and you can tell if the space is filled in and the images clear and the colors fitting, but beyond that there is something almost invisible, a haze, a vibration, a je ne sais quoi that makes all the difference. If you can perceive this finish, and more so if you can make it happen, you are close to being an artist. It could be that the difference lies entirely in the bloom. The best artists are not exactly makers, they are masters of the bloom.

To grasp the meaning of bloom, take a few lines from William Shakespeare, whose writing is all about the finish. Consider the opening of Sonnet 116:

> Let me not to the marriage of true minds
> Admit impediments; love is not love
> Which alters when it alteration finds,
> Or bends with the remover to remove.
> O no, it is an ever-fixèd mark
> That looks on tempests and is never shaken.

The ideas in this passage can change your life, but the polish of it makes you want to keep it in your heart forever. The word order alone elevates the plain sentiments into art. It could say, "Don't let me get in the way of a good marriage," but instead it allows you to think more deeply and even nobly about constancy in a marriage. You read these lines and you feel the polish bodily, taking it in, into the depths of your heart as well as your mind.

I feel the same about Thoreau's writing, both in his rougher journals and in his books, like *Walden*. He achieves the kind of finish that is not inconsistent with his life on the trail and in a boat. He has his own way of rubbing his words with wax and creating a sheen. A passage from his journal entry for August 30, 1856, reads: "Let not your life be wholly without an object, though it be only to ascertain the flavor of a cranberry, for it will not be only the quality of an insignificant berry that you will have tasted, but the flavor of your life to that extent, and it will be such a sauce as no wealth can buy."[3] This is one of the running themes in Thoreau's reflections—the experience of nature is worth far more than ordinary measures of wealth—but here there is art in the language that elevates it and gives it a finish.

This philosophy of the finish is not one widely followed in our contemporary world. We want our words to communicate a message and not necessarily to have polish. We are concerned about the basics, and yet Thoreau is reminding us that the basics do not give us the life we seek. We remain in our daily lives without a bloom, and that lack gets translated into feelings of lostness and emptiness. We know something is missing, but we assume it is a functional absence and not the loss of a blueberry's frosty glow.

Most people today would likely admit that society does not have much polish. We do not see the point in having manners or formalities. Our language is often crude, and our communications in emails and texts usually lack style. A bloom on daily discourse is not necessary, but it could humanize our relationships and take the edge off our interactions.

People ask me how to be a successful writer. I might say, "Focus on the finish," intending the pun but taking it seriously. You do both in your art and craft, especially in the art and craft of your life: Move toward a good end, but develop a talent for topping your life and work with a gorgeous bloom, like the soft ash pearl on a blueberry or the misty blue-purple fog on a mountain.

22

THE HEAVENS WITHDRAW

And now another friendship is ended. I do not know what has made my friend doubt me, but I know that in love there is no mistake, and that every estrangement is well founded. The heavens withdraw and arch themselves higher. I am sensible not only of a moral, but even a grand physical pain such as gods may feel, about my head and breast, a certain ache and fullness . . . My life is like a stream that is suddenly dammed and has no outlet; but it rises higher up the hills that shut it in, and will become a deep and silent lake . . . Undoubtedly our good genii have mutually found the material unsuitable . . . Each man or woman is a veritable god or goddess, but to the mass of their fellows disguised.[1]

—Henry David Thoreau, journal entry, February 28, 1857

In this unconventional reflection on friendship, Henry David Thoreau is talking about a temporary break in his close relationship with Ralph Waldo Emerson. Up to this point they had enjoyed an intimacy for twelve years, but it was never smooth running. Thoreau was a rough man at home in boots or in a homemade boat, and Emerson was genteel and perhaps fussy in his stately study and out in town. Emerson's contemporaries described him as modest, friendly, generous, hospitable, and even "ethereal," but his friends and even his wife Lidean called him Mr. Emerson, pointing to the formality and distance that was part of his character.

Thoreau's idea of friendship begins with the idea that it is not personal or interpersonal but is rather the work of the gods. Thoreau had received a classical education at Harvard, reading philosophy in the original Greek and translating the great playwrights. He was familiar with the centuries-long habit of artists to refer to the classical gods and goddesses as images for the basic powers of life. Respecting these gods can be somewhere between poetry and religion, taking them seriously but not as a matter of belief.

If the two men had run into a blockage, Thoreau explains that their good genii, their guiding spirits or daimons, found a problem in the materials of their relationship. Again, the genius and daimon are unnamed forces, not to be believed in but cautiously noticed. The angels of friendship and not the two men's personalities caused the temporary separation.

Thoreau sounds so twenty-first-century when he says, "In love there is no mistake." Even a rupture in affection has its place. Problems and disruptions are part of friendship and do not necessarily point to a collapse of the relationship. The gods have a better overview of what the friendship needs, and their interference, sometimes causing conflict, can be respected. They will elevate the bond in their own mysterious time and manner. "The heavens withdraw and arch themselves higher."

When we run into trouble in a relationship, we might take a larger view and understand that the heavens are withdrawing to give the intimacy greater dimension. Including the gods and goddesses is a way of transforming the narrative of the friendship into myth, the only adequate story for a friendship having the weight of Emerson and Thoreau's. Thoreau said that relationships need a poetic base, and one good poetic form is myth.

From their personal perspective, Emerson and Thoreau tried to get along, but we can see a wider, deeper aspect of their intimacy, not only as an essential American phenomenon, but as a model of human intertextuality, their unique perspectives intersecting and the will of the gods running along with the wishes of the friends.

Even the intense pain Thoreau feels at the interruption of his intimacy with Emerson is the rupture created by the gods moving around with their various purposes. The malady is more than human, even though it is felt in the human breast.

Thoreau moves to another metaphor. In the disturbance in friendship that causes so much pain, a stream is being blocked up to create a dam that will increase in depth. The friendship is ripening, and so the blockage serves a purpose. Through discomfort and temporary separation, a trickle has become a lake. What an important lesson for modern people in all their intense relationships: to allow the ups and downs for the eventual deepening of love.

Now we find that the gods or genii judge the materials of the friendship good and can proceed. What a thought! Relationship problems are a reorganization of the materials of that union. As a therapist, I have often tried to see seeds of maturing in relationship troubles. The alternate tendency is to look for behaviors that are not "working," as though friendship were a machine. Or we try to discover where we have gone wrong. We try to fix it. The real problem is that we are out of sync with the gods. Or, the gods are at work creating the desired union, and their point of view differs from ours, leading to conflicts.

Boldly, Thoreau takes a final step. The people we relate to are actually gods and goddesses in disguise. Perhaps the real friend Thoreau discovered in Emerson was Apollo, Greek god of poetry, the arts, and music. Maybe the god Emerson found in Thoreau was Pan, a nature spirit, known for his lively dance, whom Emerson loved, or even Artemis, goddess of the forest and animals and plants. I favor Artemis, because the gods do not have to fit the gender of the human, and this goddess I expect would take under her care a pure-minded, thoughtful, natural man like Thoreau. In the ancient stories Artemis often enjoyed the companionship of a young man: Orion, Acteon, Hippolytos. I like to think of Thoreau as the new Acteon, a young man who abandons his civilized farm for the forest wilderness and is transformed by what he finds there.

In his elegy for Thoreau, written just five years after this journal entry, Emerson referred to the difficulties and problems, thus being much in tune with Thoreau's own analysis that includes the gods and daimons. This was a deep friendship, one that qualifies for the term *anam cara*, the Irish phrase for a special relationship in which the people enjoy each other's company and at the same time involve themselves in their friend's struggles to navigate a good life.

Here we have essential ingredients for restoring our humanity: living more deliberately, taking each other seriously, embracing the many emotions of love, and honoring the gods and goddesses playing out within us and around us. Here psychology and natural religion come together: dealing directly with our emotions and respecting the great powers working through us.

There is a tendency today to make all of this psychology, where the gods are *parts* of us. But that is exactly the wrong direction. The gods may be disguised as human factors in relationship, but they are not human. They are other. And this separation allows Thoreau to speak of the genii approving or not the materials of the friendship. This way of granting our emotions their transcendence helps us deal with the grating powers of love and individual integrity and makes for a vastly layered and profound human life.

23

I AM STONE

I am the nature of stone. It takes the summer's sun to warm it. My acquaintances sometimes imply that I am too cold; but each thing is warm enough of its kind. Is the stone too cold which absorbs the heat of the summer sun and does not part with it during the night? Crystals, though they be of ice, are not too cold to melt, but it was in the melting that they were formed. Cold! I am most sensible of warmth in winter days. It is not the warmth of fire that you would have, but everything is warm and cold according to its nature. It is not that I am too cold, but that our warmth and coldness are not of the same nature; hence when I am absolutely warmest, I may be coldest to you. Crystal does not complain of crystal any more than the dove of its mate. You who complain that I am cold find Nature cold. To me she is warm. My heat is latent to you. Fire itself is cold to whatever is not of a nature to be warmed by it. A cool wind is warmer to a feverish man that the air of a furnace. That I am cold means that I am of another nature.[1]

—Henry David Thoreau, journal entry, December 21, 1851

This rhapsody on cold says something about the freedom to be who and what you are and not to adjust to the expectations of others, who are not of the same emotional temperature as you. What is warm to you might be cold to someone else. Your cold is yours and cannot be shared with others who have their own kind of cold. And, a person who is by nature warm, may not experience your coldness in the way that you do.

Henry David Thoreau was cold in some ways, although from this journal entry we understand that he did not think of himself as being cold. Emotionally cold, that is. Others might experience him as cold since they had their own experience and definitions of cold. He is of the nature of stone, he writes, that takes a summer sun to warm it. These two qualities, cold and stone, and maybe stone cold, are alchemical aspects of a person, elements in their makeup. Most people would probably rather not be described by these words, but Thoreau just accepted them as facts. He is stone and he is cold. It takes special conditions and time to make a stone warm.

Alchemists felt that stone was a valuable quality, offering substance, toughness, and endurance. In fact, they referred to the goal of alchemical procedures as achieving the stone, the *lapis philosophorum*, the philosopher's stone. This was not stone as we know it, as when we come across it on a hike. This is the stone that lies in every atom of your body and soul. It defines you, and when people encounter you, they meet your cold stone, not just your surface personality. If you have the solidity of stone in your character, cold may naturally accompany it. Coldness may be related to personal substance, as it seems to have been in Thoreau.

Obviously, Thoreau did not have a sentimental idea of himself as being soft and warm and sweet. On the contrary, he was tough, realistic, and sometimes cool. In spite of these qualities, many people loved him. They felt the warmth in his cold character and understood the paradoxes that Thoreau presents in this journal entry. Notice that it is from December 21, the first day of winter that year.

People in the United States tend to be warm on the outside and cool inwardly. Visitors often remark on the way Americans smile all the time, and yet they are not always welcoming. On many occasions I have lived in Ireland, where people are also warm, not like Yanks, but in their own welcoming way. Yet I know that the smile and good humor can spin around in a flash, and then you will see penetrating judgment and argument. People around the world are cool and warm in national ways, as slight differences in emotional temperature define a national character.

It is not easy sometimes to see that for others warm is cold and cold is preferable. Reading his journals, you see that Thoreau enjoyed cold weather and didn't mind having a cool temperament, which he felt was warmer than the warmth he felt in others. But it was not just a matter of warm in some being cool in others, but that warm can be cool and cool warm, depending on the person.

One writer devoted to Antarctica relates this experience: "I remember quite vividly, having been in Antarctica for nearly a year, when the supply ship came in on what we considered a balmy day. We winterers were walking around in t-shirts and loose un-tucked over shirts with rolled up sleeves, while those who were new arrivals were well wrapped in fastened jackets and hats and still feeling cold. The two groups surveyed each other with some puzzlement."[2]

This, of course, takes cold literally, but the same might be said about emotional coldness. Some people regard each other with some puzzlement. The warm ones don't understand and may not accept cold, and vice versa. Thoreau would be in the group of winterers and the people in his circle more sensitive to the cold. Imagine walking into a group of people knowing the relativity of warm and cold and not being so offended by those who enjoy a colder inner climate.

On our general point of learning from Thoreau how to be more deeply human, we might hesitate to dismiss someone because we sense coldness in him. Cold is one of the qualities of human life, like one of the ancient humors. Some of us have more of this humor, some less, and it may determine what kind of person we are. We may have a touch of cold and a touch of warm. Thoreau asks us to see the benefit in that touch and not demand that everyone have the same quantities and qualities of hot and cold.

As a psychotherapist, I value any power in me to remain cool in circumstances when emotions are high. I don't want to be judged as a cold person, but I assume that my clients appreciate the cool climate I can bring at times to our important conversations. My cool is not without its warmth anyway, since my overall attitude toward my client is based on friendship. At times, we all need to keep cool and appear cold, even if we are temperamentally warm.

Thoreau lived close to the natural world and appreciated its sometimes cold heart. It may have been the cold waters of Walden Pond that lowered his emotional temperature and allowed him to see life from his cool point of view. But we might remember here that Henry's brother John died from tetanus when Henry was in his twenties. Soon after, Henry developed John's symptoms. It was not a cold person who identified spontaneously with his brother's torments.

Thoreau shows us how to value the underappreciated in life—in this case, the cool emotions—and reevaluate these qualities. He also helps us see life's subtleties, the warmth in the cool and the chill in warmth. The goal in most things is not only to appreciate opposites, but to see how they live in each other.

24

LAPSE OF TIME

Often I can give the truest and most interesting account of any adventure I have had after years have elapsed, for then I am not confused, only the most significant facts surviving in my memory. Indeed, all that continues to interest me after such a lapse of time is sure to be pertinent, and I may safely record all that I remember.[1]

—Henry David Thoreau, journal entry, March 28, 1857

Once again Henry David Thoreau turns the world upside down. We often try to put down our recollection of an event soon after it happens, when it is fresh in our minds. Here he says we can give the truest account after years have elapsed. How can that be? And does this say anything important about memory, storytelling, or a sense of self?

Early memories seem to be recordings of things that happened to us, but, as we remember the facts, our mind strays to timeless essentials. An event happened in my childhood on a certain day, but that event says something about childhood itself and maybe about me at any age. In memory I find my absolute self and uncover things about me that are not conditioned by time. I also learn much about what a child is, and I may come to realize that the spirit of the child, its essence, stays with me my whole life. I may need some distance on the facts to understand how deep and long my memories are fixed.

Thoreau says that there is a kind of winnowing process that takes place over time. "Only the most significant facts survive in my memory." When I tell a story from my distant past, my story may be true and interesting because certain details have risen to the top. What is important in the story has become obvious over time. Early on I didn't know which details would prove central. But now I know, and now I can tell a better story about events. Now I may *safely* record my impressions.

Here we get a hint that the factual recording of an event doesn't give us as much information as a thoughtful reconstruction of it over time, in the emergence of a real story. Eventually we learn what is truly important in the story, and then our narrative offers a deeper understanding of the events.

I have a story from my life that I have written about several times. I was a university professor, loving the work and the setting. I assumed I would do that work for the rest of my life, but one day the head of my department told me that the faculty met and decided to let me go, not to give me tenure.

This was one of the shocking moments of my life, because I thought I was doing a good job and giving my all to teaching. I was disappointed, to say the least, and didn't know what I would do next. It so happened that people then began asking me to be their psychotherapist, and soon I was able to get a license and open a private practice. I survived quite well, although ever since, I have missed teaching at a university. I have hoped over the years that some institution would offer me a position.

I used to tell this story with the feeling of disbelief that the original faculty didn't recognize my contributions. But over time, I began to see that they were a conservative group, and my approach to my field of religious studies was unconventional. I could have taught it with a little more tradition, and my approach may have been understood. I notice something unsettling in my nature: I often go my own way and disregard traditions that have their value. In many areas this tendency, perhaps a runaway spirit of youth, has limited my impact. I now see all of this from a distance, and I think Thoreau was right: I can only understand this story of rejection much later.

We could do our cultural history from a distance, too. When we are so close to events we do not see deeper and larger patterns. We see facts, but we fail to notice the deep mythic images and episodes that tell us what is really happening below the surface. We do not see the underlying sagas and episodes that reveal meaning. We see real people but fail to see the fingers and faces of fairy tales and songs and riddles. Is the past that we so easily romanticize a recalling of Eden, a time both pristine and perfect?

Historians tell us what happened, but because they are so serious and precise they fail to notice the figures of fairy tales, myths, and even movies that reveal the deeper narratives. It requires some distance to glimpse the imaginal and detect the mythological. Perhaps Thoreau is telling us to take our time and allow the invisibles to manifest.

Future generations may reveal what we have done and who we are. We are too close to the action and think too seriously that we know what we are doing and what it is all about. What is invisible in our world today may finally show itself to our children, who will in good humor forgive us for being so dense about our own actions and understandings.

One day people will know all those important things we did not see as we went about our lives and tried to figure ourselves out. There is an ocean of debris created by our busyness and in the depth of it lie the underlying storylines that we were trying to work out. Call it our unconscious, or the id, or the collective flotsam that is revealed over time.

Thoreau is hinting, as a proto Sigmund Freud, that there is a vast element in us that we know little about, but if we dig away at it we will see it and then understand who we are and what our life project is. Our stories of the past tell us how the psyche works and who we are at the deepest level. They can be read and heard archetypally, as revealing our essence. They reveal the causes of our present behavior because they show us the narratives and patterns that are always there shaping experience.

Depth psychology tells us that memories of childhood are not about childhood but about the essential idea of child or the eternal child. This approach goes against common sense as much as Thoreau's idea does and could be closely related. The stories we tell, even our histories, are not so much about what happened as about what happens. They tell us how life is, not just how it was. Our stories are more philosophical than historical. They give us the mysteries of life, which is more than a surface chronicle of events. If we wait long enough, our remembered stories will reveal the secrets of our existence.

25

IMPORTED WOODS

When we walk, we naturally go to the fields and woods: what would become of us, if we walked only in a garden or a mall? Even some sects of philosophers have felt the necessity of importing the woods to themselves, since they did not go to the woods. "They planted groves and walks of Platanes [sycamore trees]," where they took subdiales ambulationes in porticos open to the air. Of course, it is of no use to direct our steps to the woods, if they do not carry us thither. I am alarmed when it happens that I have walked a mile into the woods bodily, without getting there in spirit. . . . The thought of some work will run in my head, and I am not where my body is, I am out of my senses. In my walks I would fain return to my senses. What business have I in the woods, if I am thinking of something out of the woods?

If you are ready to leave father and mother, and brother and sister, and wife and child and friends, and never see them again?—if you have paid your debts, and made your will, and settled all your affairs, and are a free man, then you are ready for a walk.[1]

—Henry David Thoreau, "Walking"

The transcendentalists of New England were incredibly dedicated walkers. They undertook prodigious walks that were long, animated by conversation and milestones in important relationships: Ralph Waldo Emerson and Nathaniel Hawthorne, Henry David Thoreau and William Ellery Channing, Hawthorne and Margaret Fuller, Thoreau in Maine and New Hampshire. For them walking was a spiritual practice equal to any spiritual exercise or monkish rite. They were devoted to walking.

Most of us probably believe that we think better when we take a walk or have good conversations while walking with a friend. There is even an ancient school of philosophy connected with Aristotle in which the thinkers, according to tradition, walked as they thought—the peripatetics. Virginia Woolf thought along the line of Thoreau and wrote, "She loves rambling alone in her woods. She loves going out by herself at night. She loves hiding from callers. She loves walking among her trees and musing."

Thoreau loved to walk among the trees while musing and thought it nothing to walk from Concord to Boston, about sixteen miles. His friend Emerson was also a walking thinker, who famously took a walk with Hawthorne in September 1842 that lasted two days. In his journal he ends his tale of the walk with a few spirited words: "From the Shaker Village we came to Littleton, & thence to Acton, still in the same redundance of splendour. It was like a day of July, and from Acton we sauntered leisurely homeward to finish the nineteen miles of our second day before four in the afternoon."[2]

Thoreau liked the word *saunter*, and at the opening of his essay on walking he offers his personalized etymology of the word, saying that it comes from la Sainte Terre, the Holy Land. "Those who never go to the Holy Land in their walks, as they pretend, are indeed mere idlers and vagabonds, but they who do go there are saunterers in the good sense, such as I mean." Emerson remembers reaching the Holy Land in his walk with Hawthorne, and similarly Thoreau's many accounts of his wanderings suggest the immeasurable rewards of his walks. He even has scruples about going into the woods in body only, leaving his spirit behind.

Walking takes on special meaning in religious contexts, such as processions, pilgrimages, and cloister walks. Even ordinary walks can have a holy purpose, like a walk around a family farm or a walk to visit an elderly relative. The family may go on a holiday hike or you may take children for an adventure. We would only have to expand and deepen our understanding of what is holy to see the sacred nature of intentional walking.

Some walks have a more mundane purpose and do not address the needs of the soul. We are there in body only and therefore lose the spiritual quality of our action, like Thoreau going into the forest without his spirit. In general, for an activity to be *religious*, in an existential and immediate sense of the word, not just conforming to a special creed or tradition, it is conscious and full of intention and care.

If you are going into the woods, it should really be a forest and not just a copse of trees or a planted grove. This does not mean that there isn't value in creating a garden or a cloister, but for Thoreau wildness is a necessity.

In the ancient Greek experience, the woods are the haunt of the goddess Artemis, and it is she that you will encounter as you move deep among the trees and away from civilization. The Greeks might also expect you to find Aphrodite in a garden or maybe Saturn in a shaded grove. The world is populated with gods and goddesses, and our excursions into it may aim at specific spiritual rewards. Again, intention and purpose count.

What Thoreau says about the woods could also apply to gardens and parks. If you enter them bodily but without a thought-out purpose, to ease yourself away from the busyness of life, samsara if you like, you may not have the full experience of a garden or portico. The same could apply to a park in the city. Pars pro toto, the park represents or embodies the forest. It is an appeal to Artemis, the deep spirit of retreat. You probably go to a park to get away from the streets and commerce, a noble motive, but you could do it with a heightened intelligence. Go for water, trees, quiet, or small animal life, and make these an inward, reviving experience.

Today you see many people running through parks with headphones on and with no obvious attention to the surroundings. Running, especially this self-absorbed kind, is not walking. When you walk, you notice the world around you and take it in, and you talk to the person you are with. Conversation is part of the walk. You are not escaping, you are becoming more engaged.

The ancient Greeks had an answer to the issue of making a park instead of entering a forest. They referred to the spirit of a smaller patch of nature as a nymph, an important part of Greek life. When we hear of nymphs, we think of a lovely figure on a rock or in the grass. But a nymph is the actual spirit of place that you can sense clearly. It is not a physical body but a strong presence, as when you stand at the edge of the ocean and sense the spirit there that you find nowhere else. The Greeks named that spirit an Oceanid, a particular kind of nymph proper to the ocean. I live among nymphs of the pond, and you might be close to river or small stream nymphs. These presences are necessary for the nourishment of your soul, and without them you shrivel up with the loss of your humanity.

You probably know when you need an Oceanid, and so you go to a beach. In general, a nymph is encountered near springs and wells, streams and pools, rivers and ponds. We go to these places not for a literal purpose, not to fill a pail with water, but to receive the spirit of the place. A nymph, the genius of a place, is its resident spirit, that can enliven a human being and give it food that keeps you alive and thriving as a person. Humans need these different kinds of spirit and quite properly visit the sea, or the desert, or a mountain, depending on what they sense is needed. When you hear someone say, "Let's go to the beach," you are getting a message from the land of the nymph, a message that expresses an essential need.

Because of our materialistic bias, the limited vision our science offers us, we fail to appreciate the importance of the spirit of a river or a pond. We feel it and may want to be near it, but we do not know intellectually how to make it an essential part of our lives. We are unconscious as we do our best to receive its gifts, and in that regard our ancient ancestors were so much more sophisticated. They named and personified these essential spirits, which made any encounter with them immediate, felt, and treasured.

Thoreau was able to restore the ancient consciousness about plants and bodies of water and creatures. He had his own vernacular language for this essential practice, as when he insisted that the muskrat was his cousin and when he invited birds to land on his shoulders. There is no reason why we could not do the same and restore our acquaintance with the nymphs, the spirits of place, who enchant streams and ponds and fill the heart with earthy but highly spiritual pleasures.

26

THE BROWS OF THE EARTH

It is worth the while to see the mountains in the horizon once a day. I have thus seen some earth which corresponds to my least earthly and trivial, to my most heavenward-looking, thoughts. The earth seen through an azure, an ethereal, veil. They are the natural temples, elevated brows, of the earth, looking at which, the thoughts of the beholder are naturally elevated and sublimed,—etherealized. I wish to see the earth through the medium of much air or heaven, for there is no paint like the air. Mountains thus seen are worthy of worship.

—Henry David Thoreau, journal
entry, September 12, 1851

They who simply climb to the peak of Monadnock have seen but little of the mountain. I came not to look off from it, but to look at it . . . The great charm is not to look off from a height, but to walk over this novel and wonderful rock surface.[1]

—Henry David Thoreau, journal
entry, August 9, 1860

I live at the foot of Mount Monadnock, in New Hampshire, a mountain that Henry David Thoreau visited several times. He described how over one hundred people might climb it in a day, and even now my family watch as many people walk the mountain's trails in all seasons. Thoreau once camped on the top with his friend Harrison Gray Otis Blake, and we had a friend who camped there once overnight. In the morning, he said, dozens of people were walking around his tent. Mount Monadnock means "The Mountain That Stands Alone," but it is never alone.

We watch this sprawling mountain from our breakfast window, as it appears and disappears in the fog and clouds. A few years ago, the local town announced a meeting for people to discuss the spiritual meaning of the mountain. Organizers were expecting a few to a dozen people to show up, but almost one hundred turned out and had a vigorous conversation. People know intuitively that mountains have a spiritual potency, and Thoreau simply touched that sensibility in the beautifully crafted paragraph quoted above.

He says we should gaze at a mountain once a day. It is a spiritual prescription, like taking an aspirin each day for your heart, only here you gaze at a mountain for your soul and spirit. Before discovering Thoreau's remarkable way of living on the planet, I was moved by the writings of Marsilio Ficino (1433–1499), a philosopher who taught similar wisdom in Florence. He said that if you're feeling sad, you should walk by a body of water sparkling in the sun. He would have liked Thoreau's similar prescription of gazing at a mountain every day.

Thoreau refers to mountains as "natural temples." We know that he was not inclined to attend church, in a place and time when churchgoing was almost universally approved and even expected. He preferred the natural holy places he could see with his naturally sanctifying eyes. He claimed to have seen angels swooping over Walden Pond, so it wasn't unusual for him to imagine mountains as natural temples.

Now, consider if we twenty-first-century people saw the sacred nature of mountains and everything on those mountains—trees, shrubs, birds, squirrels, and rocks—as sacred, we might be motivated to protect and nurture those holy things. The neglect of nature begins with the secularization of life, with the loss of a sense of the holy in the world. The point, Thoreau says, is to walk those rocky surfaces and behold them by means of the heavenly vision we have discovered from their heights. Mountains take our focus upward, where we sense intuitively that the sacred resides. When we pray, we naturally lift our heads upward in quiet hope, if not downward in meditative silence.

Here is a clue to restoring our humanity. Human beings need close family life, intimate relationships, a cozy home, and good home-cooked meals, but we also benefit from the sight of soaring mountains and a view of the sky and the feel of ascension under our feet as we climb upward. We need grand vision and hope and adventure. These are goals that we glimpse in the sight of mountains, because ascending is never only physical. The sheer sight of a high mountain teaches us about going high in our lives and in our thoughts. Climbing a mountain can be an instructive poetic and spiritual experience.

Ralph Waldo Emerson, Nathaniel Hawthorne, and Thoreau made their way slowly to Mount Monadnock from Concord, Massachusetts, with thoughts of possibility and purity and, full of intention, climbed this mountain that I see every day. Thoreau was heading to a natural temple on a pilgrimage to be lifted up, a goal that no doubt motivates many pilgrims to visit or climb many holy mountains in the world. He suggested not going to the top for a panoramic view, although Emerson, perhaps the more spiritual of the pair, described the many ponds and farms he saw from the crest of Monadnock. Thoreau did not want to conquer a mountain, but rather to be raised in thought and sensibility by means of it. "They who simply climb to the peak of Monadnock have seen but little of the mountain," he wrote. Therefore, logically, they have been elevated in spirit only a little.

Mountains can also be dangerous to the soul. The hero obtains satisfaction from getting to the top and conquering a challenge rather than taking it in and becoming a deeper person in the midst of it. Thoreau's approach would be a tonic and maybe even a cure for this modern anxiety disorder by which many measure themselves by whether they have overcome nature or want to be in it.

This modest, incidental teaching by Thoreau could change modern life for the better and could be applied in politics, business, and other areas. Instead of conquering cancer, we could get to know it better and apply emotions of care, concern, and depth analysis. We could even learn from it how to live and maybe eventually be freed of its deathly claim on us. Instead of focusing mainly on self-interest in politics, we could work for the advancement of the system of government, the citizens, and the people of the world. We do not have to go up to the top of the mountain and feel justified for having won and conquered. We do not need thrills as much as we need self-transformation and deep satisfaction.

With Thoreau, we could be *in* the mountain enjoying its essence rather than on top, feeling heroic as we gaze at the world spreading around and beneath us. When you have the feeling that other people are beneath you, in any situation, you are in the area of ego, not soul. This lesson also shows us how to read Thoreau and be instructed by his special genius: His subtle observations of nature and its ways show us how best to be human.

Thoreau asks us to look at every aspect of our lives "through an azure, an ethereal, veil." It is like having glasses or filters the color of the blue sky, taking it all metaphorically, of course, having the highest values and interpretations of lowly life. For example, parents wishing to do a good job of raising a child could reflect on the role of parenthood in the largest and most ideal context, instead of doing it unconsciously or only according to the way they were brought up. The azure veil takes you to the most pristine and exalted ways of seeing all your roles in life, especially one as crucial as orienting a child in life.

Look at a mountain every day as a prescription for the health of your soul. If you don't have a mountain nearby, have a good painting or photo of a mountain in your home for your daily contemplation. Make this your mantra: I will not climb too high in anything I do. I will remain in the thick of life, while ascending, absorbing its wisdom.

27

THE MUSIC OF THE WORLD

Thoreau's sister Helen died of tuberculosis, and later ministers performed the funeral in the parlor of the Thoreau house. At the end of the funeral, Thoreau "stood to wind a music box to the tune of the sweetest tenderest minor strains that seemed like no earthly tune. All sat quietly until it was through." Amanda Mathers Recollections of Thoreau, Thoreau Society Bulletin.[1]

—Laura Dassow Walls, *Thoreau: A Life*

What is there in music that it should so stir our deeps? We are all ordinarily in a state of desperation, such is our life; oftimes it drives us to suicide. . . . But let us hear certain strains of music, we are at once advertised of a life which no man has told us of, which no preacher preaches. . . . We are actually lifted above ourselves.[2]

—Henry David Thoreau,
journal entry, January 15, 1857

When my hoe tinkled against the stones, that music echoed to the woods and the sky and was an accompaniment to my labor which yielded an instant and immeasurable crop. . . . I remembered with as much pity as pride, if I remembered at all, my acquaintances who had gone to the city to attend the oratorios.[3]

—Henry David Thoreau, *Walden*

Went into the woods by Holden Swamp and sat down to hear the wind roar amid the tree-tops . . . It is a music that wears better than the opera, methinks. This reminds me how the telegraph wire hummed coarsely in the tempest as we passed under it.[4]

—Henry David Thoreau, journal entry, November 9, 1853

The commonest and cheapest sounds as the barking of a dog, produce the same effect on fresh and healthy ears that the rarest music does . . . I have lain awake at night many a time to think of the barking of a dog which I had heard long before, bathing my being again in those waves of sound, as a frequenter of the opera might lie awake remembering the music he had heard.[5]

—Henry David Thoreau, *Walden*

It seemed by the distant hum as if somebody's bees had swarmed, and that the neighbors, according to Virgil's advice, by a faint tintinnabulum upon the most sonorous of their domestic utensils, were endeavoring to call them down into the hive again.[6]

—Henry David Thoreau, *Walden*

I sit in my boat on Walden, playing the flute this evening, and see the perch, which I seem to have charmed, hovering around me, and the moon traveling over the bottom, which is strewn with the wrecks of the forest, and feel that nothing but the wildest imagination can conceive of the manner of life we are living. Nature is a wizard. The Concord nights are stranger than the Arabian Nights.[7]

—Henry David Thoreau, journal entry, May 27, 1841

Henry David Thoreau liked to play his flute out in the wild, the instrument of the god Pan who danced the wild step of life in ancient, mythic Arcadia, a wilderness area of Greece and a common image for natural life. The ancient *Homeric Hymn to Pan* could be a psalm in honor of Thoreau:

In the evening Pan returns from the hunt with a shout
and then plays gentle music on his reeds.
He is better than the bird that perches among the leaves
in flowery springtime
and sends off his sad song with honey-soaked tones.
The musical mountain nymphs join him,
dancing with fast movements and singing next to a dark spring,
as echoes scream about the mountaintop.
The nature spirit floats here and there and then right into the dance,
taking the lead with his quick feet.
He has a lynxskin on his back
as he gives himself joyfully to the piercing songs
in the quiet meadow where the crocus and aromatic hyacinth
bloom and mingle intimately with the grass.

> *They sing of the holy gods and goddesses*
> *and the celestial Olympus.*[8]

Thoreau heard music in his daily brush with the world: in the ding of a hoe and the barking of a dog. You may find aesthetic pleasure at the echoing ring of a thin goblet or the shuffle of a shoe. Remarkable sounds are all around us and a person devoted to nature might well hear music everywhere.

In the sixth century C.E., the philosopher Boethius compared *musica humana*, the rhythms of emotions or stages in life, to *musica mundana*, world music, the passing of seasons and the percussion of rain. *Musica instrumentalis*, the art of music we hear in concerts and through headphones, offers an aesthetic representation of the world's natural music. Thoreau was a musica mundana specialist who often contrasted the earthy thing-music he loved with a Boston performance, preferring the music of the world.

This odd way of seeing things may seem merely quaint and charming, but it offers a serious idea about living on our planet. The ground of our daily lives is not a physical platform, like a flat wooden stage, but an aesthetic and artistic place in which we are elevated to high level of participation. The world is full of artistic expression that is not the creative work of humans but an offshoot of organic processes. Our planet is not only a well-functioning orb but also has artistic powers offering an infinite variety of sounds and visual images. We note this aesthetic when we comment gratefully on the beauty of a sunset and notice the artistic lure of the sound of rushing water.

The various arts of nature, like music, are forever appealing to our senses, but we often fail to look or listen. We become absorbed in the utility and economics of life around us. We are more interested in how the world works than in how it expresses itself beautifully. Thoreau never embraced natural science fully because he enjoyed the music of the natural world more than its measured and quantified profiles.

"We are actually lifted above ourselves," says Thoreau. He often uses the word *elevate*. Human beings need to be lifted because naturally—that is, unconsciously—we are thickheaded and heavy-handed, going about our lower business without thought of evolving into something greater. The arts in general have the power to lift us up to another level of existence, while the arts of nature show us how to live spiritually.

Thoreau goes on to say that this is a marvelous world we live in, stranger than the Arabian Nights with all its enchantment. What inspires this comment? The perch who appear from deep in the water at the sound of tintinnabulum on Thoreau's flute. Thoreau was a powerful orphic musician and magician, charming nature with his instrument. Pan incarnated.

This transcendentalist theory of music fits into Thoreau's general approach to life, especially life in the natural world. To go up, you must go down. You go deep into the muddy, wet, and slimy realm of rivers and mountain trails to find your higher humanity and your deepest identity. You discover that music, like the other arts, is magical, not in a broad metaphorical sense, but because of its capacity to charm animals and lift humans to their higher natures. Music is not merely entertaining. It has potency. Thoreau rejects the oratorios one could listen to in Boston, and he presents an alternative: the sonorities of ordinary life.

In my youth, I studied music composition seriously with a few genius composers. Along the way, I got interested in nature music as a part of my classical style of writing. I brought recording devices out into fields and brought home the sounds of waterfalls and blowing leaves and inserted them into my music. Now my daughter, a professional musician, also includes the sounds of nature in her impressive albums. So, I would not make the distinction Thoreau makes between his hoe clinking at Walden and the oratorios being performed in Boston. They are two related ways of lifting humanity out of its lower nature into its promise.

Life is musical, with its high notes and low notes, its themes and variations, and its intros and codas. The sounds of our instruments merely echo and emulate the music of the world, allowing us to enjoy the pure form of sound without any complicating counterpoints from life. In *Walden*, Thoreau said he walked through the gossips of the village with his thoughts on higher things, like Orpheus singing the praises of the gods. Orpheus is a good myth to link to Thoreau. Both could charm animals and both liked to play their musical instruments, lyre and flute, respectively, in the forest.

Thoreau's natural music also reveals his process, the way he thinks and works. He goes into nature and is aware of its messages, the soft ways it reveals its secrets. From his long hours on a river or walking farmlands and forests he learns life's mysteries and immediately applies them to his own life. Therefore, his writings present us with the natural world but also with nature's guidance about how to live. Deep in the woods you do not become a feral creature, you become a cultured one in whom the natural world is contained in human form.

An artist's sensitivity could make a better world, for the perception of beauty makes a person sensitive to the environment. At every turn we could listen for the world's music and relate to that world more sensually and intimately. With Thoreau's simple aesthetics, as I write my books, I pound away at my computer keyboard and enjoy the muted percussion of its keys. Everything has its own music if you have the ear for it.

28

DRIED FUNGUS

I wish to thank you again for those books. They are the nucleus of my library . . . The books have long been shelved in cases of my own construction made partly of the driftwood of our river. They are the admiration of all beholders. Alcott and Emerson, besides myself have been cracking some of the nuts.

Certainly I shall never pay you for them. Of those new to me the Rig Veda is the most savory that I have yet tasted. As primitive poetry, I think as any extant. Indeed all the Vedantic literature is priceless . . . I shall browse there for some winters to come . . .

I have just taken a run up country, as I did with you once, only a little farther this time, to the Connecticut river in New Hampshire, where I saw Alcott, King of men. He is among those who ask after you, and takes a special interest in the oriental books. He cannot say enough about them.

I am sorry that I can give but a poor account of myself. I got "run down" they say, more than a year ago, and have not yet got fairly up again. It has not touched my spirits however, for they are as indifferently tough, as sluggishly resilient, as a dried

> *fungus. I would it were the kind called punk, that they might catch and retain some heavenly spark.*[1]
>
> —Henry David Thoreau to Thomas Cholmondeley, October 20, 1856

Thomas Cholmondeley (pronounced "Chumley") was an English gentleman who visited Henry David Thoreau, staying at his family's Concord house for a fall season, where they became good friends. Later, Cholmondeley sent Thoreau a gift of forty-four volumes of Eastern writings, including the Rig Veda, the Bhagavad Gita, and the Upanishads. Thoreau knew most of that literature but was overjoyed to have the set in his room, a treasure on the driftwood bookshelves he had made.

In his letter he makes the point that his friends, including Ralph Waldo Emerson and Bronson Alcott, were interested in the books, giving us a peek into the literary taste of the transcendentalists. Thoreau says that he woke up the morning after he unpacked the books and melted with pleasure at the sight of them. This is the man known for his extravagant and thoughtful walking and rough boating and for classifying the many plants and trees in and around his hometown of Concord, Massachusetts. He was good at mingling mind and body.

It would be good for Earth's future if some of the basic ideas of the East became better known. I cannot imagine my life and work without the Tao, Emptiness, the Four Noble Truths, Quan Yin's compassion, or the Prajnaparamita perfection of wisdom. For me, Eastern articulations of insight are not interesting options in making sense of life. They are essential and offer necessary foundations for a philosophy of life. For many years, I have had a plan to spend my later years studying the Sanskrit language so I can read some of those great writings in the original language.

Ideas in general are not just facts and definitions but a form of imagination and a way of living internally. They can feed your soul by giving you tools for exploring the subtle workings of life and the building blocks of reflection. To live fully we need both to live with some intensity and to consider life deeply. But many people have not been introduced to this rule of life, and their brains get tired when faced with multilayered thought or obscure language. Similarly, politicians face profound issues of life and culture, but often they are not prepared to enter the required realm of rich ideas. In their grand speeches there may be little exploration of revealing thoughts and surely not many references to ancient teachings from the East. This omission is a real loss, because we need Eastern concepts to deal with life effectively.

Ideas are tied to their places of origin. Just as the art of Africa introduces forms and practices not found elsewhere and are therefore enriching, ideas and language from the Orient provide unusual ways of navigating life and interpreting the universe. Anyone might benefit from exposure to Indian, Chinese, and Japanese ideas. We have not yet adequately mined non-Western insights from Africa, Australia, New Zealand, and South America. One can only imagine what it will be like to have literature arriving from other planets. If they should come in my lifetime, I will imitate Thoreau and build some driftwood shelving.

The image of Thoreau waking to the joyous sight of forty-four volumes of Eastern writings adds a lesson for us as we attempt to elevate the human condition. Certainly, if we admired and treasured the writings of another culture, our thinking would not only benefit from new information but from new modes of thinking and for establishing humanizing values.

I understand why Thoreau and his friends treasured literature from the East so much. I find a near-perfect mode of theology there, treating divinity with strong devotion but without the personalism that has been so much part of Western spirituality. Sometimes I can express my highest ideals only in the language of the East. We would all benefit from having a few Zen, Taoism, and Buddhism volumes in our homes, and what a world we would have if everyone were as excited as Thoreau about a gift of the Rig Veda.

At the end of the aforementioned passage, Thoreau sinks into his familiar funk, although he claims resilience. He wishes he had punk in him, a fungus used to start celestial fires. He would like an uplifting spark to sustain him in times of illness. Being close to nature every day gave him grounding and basics, but he also needed intellectual kindling, ideas that would keep his creative work alive.

Thoreau's goal was to live essentially and not superficially. Since he tended toward self-effacement and discouragement, he needed guidance and a constant source of ideas. He found them especially in the Bhagavad Gita, the Upanishads, and other Eastern writings. More than once in his journals he says that he is a yogi, and he repeatedly claimed that Walden waters were identical with the Ganges River. All water is holy, and that realization puts new meaning in the boating that was so central in his life.

In spite of appearances, Thoreau never boated on the actual Assabet and Concord Rivers, because when he did so he knew he was actually on the Ganges and the Euphrates Rivers. I wish I could convey this truth adequately: To live with our full humanity we could imagine the mythological in every instance of the actual. A meaningful life depends on the ability to sense the mythic and the sacred in the most mundane and nearby presentations of nature. You never swim in a lake or ocean, because every body of water, no matter how mundane and familiar, is more importantly a representation of the Ganges, the Rivers of Paradise, and the Jordan River of Jesus's time.

29

ORGANIC EARTH

There is motion in the earth as well as on the surface; it lives and grows. It is warmed and influenced by the sun, just as my blood by my thought. I seem to see some of the life that is in the sleeping bud and blossom more intimately, nearer its fountainhead, the fancy sketches and designs of the artist. It is more simple and primitive growth; as if for ages sand and clay might have thus flowed into the forms of foliage, before plants were produced to clothe the earth. The earth I tread on is not a dead, inert mass. It is a body, has a spirit, is organic, and fluid to the influence of its spirit, and to whatever particle of that spirit is in me. She is not dead, but sleepeth. . . . Even the solid globe is permeated by the living law. It is the most living of creatures. No doubt all creatures that live on its surface are but parasites.[1]

—Henry David Thoreau, journal entry, December 31, 1851

Henry David Thoreau spent his days in the forest, set aside his books on botany, and learned that Earth is the most living of creatures. James Lovelock, who came up with the Gaia hypothesis in the 1970s, a scientific view of the planet as an organism, faced strong criticism for contradicting Charles Darwin's natural selection theory and for Gaia's similarity to certain religious and spiritual cosmologies. Like Lovelock, Thoreau did not cave in to the materialist science that could have saved his reputation and given him a place in the modern movement to dissect nature. He kept reductionistic materialism out of his natural science, leaving room for his discovery of nature's soul, as well as the divinity he believed was always hidden deep within the natural world. Nor as a lover of nature did he hide his mysticism.

As Thoreau pictures the universe, the sun warms the planet just the way it warms his body, keeping it alive and healthy, and the planet is of the same nature as his body. Looking at the universe this way, he could see life in plants and trees "more intimately." His gaze came nearer to the source of the world and his own existence. He did not speak of a creator but looked at the natural world and saw himself as a body part, maybe a parasite.

Both Thoreau and Ralph Waldo Emerson read the Neoplatonists, philosophers like Plotinus, Iamblichus, and Porphyry, who, though philosophers, were also mystics. It was there they may have found the idea of a world soul. In his Divinity School address, Emerson said plainly that what is needed in our increasingly shallow religious forms is "soul, soul, and more soul."[2] The Neoplatonists had cultivated the idea of anima mundi, the world's soul, which in Emerson is the oversoul.

Thoreau echoes William Blake, William Morris, and other practicing Neoplatonists when he writes: "It is the marriage of the soul with nature that makes the intellect fruitful and gives birth to imagination." If there was anything in the bedrock of Thoreau's life thinking it was his ability to let imagination penetrate everything, even as he walked through the woods and kept his eyes down toward the water when he paddled the rivers.

As he toured his world, Thoreau's imagination transmuted it bit by bit. He saw the earth as a living organism not through scientific analysis, as Lovelock did, but through his direct experience of the local environment. He does not have to show how the planet works as an organism but to heed the imagination as it does its work. Paddling the rivers and camping in the mountains was Thoreau's way of knowing nature. His daily life in nature colored his way of understanding that world.

When I was in my mid-thirties and completing my doctoral studies in religion, I came across the writings and practices of a Neoplatonist in fifteenth-century Florence: Marsilio Ficino. In those days I could not find much scholarship on Ficino, and so I had to make a translation of my own of his most penetrating work, *De Vita Coelitus Comparanda* (*Designing Your Life in Accord with the Sky*), a book on the soul that draws its wisdom from traditional astrology and from Arabic twists found in the writing of al-Kindī. As I was struggling with Renaissance Latin, I came across this startling statement, "The world itself is an animal, more uniquely than any other animal, and in a way the most perfect animal."[3]

I wondered if maybe it was a typo, of which there were many in the manuscripts. Maybe the word was *anima* (soul), not *animal.* But as I read further, it became clear that Ficino was speaking of the world, *mundus*, not just as a living organism, but as an animal. Imagine the planet not just having animals on it, and not just being alive, but an animal itself. This image of our planet could transform the way we live.

Neoplatonism is a philosophical movement credited to the philosopher Plotinus, who lived in Alexandria, Egypt, and died in 270 C.E.

A passage from Plotinus that applies to Thoreau's perspective reads: "This All is one universally comprehensive living being, encircling all the living beings within it, and having a soul, one soul, which extends to all is members."[4]

Clearly, Thoreau felt "encircled" by the All in nature, often recommending searching out the divine lurking in nature. In this theology, you do not need a religion to be religious. You do not need a creed or rite to be in the presence of divinity. Plotinus added that the most direct way to soul is beauty, and Thoreau, too, was drawn to nature primarily for its beauty.

All things share in the world's soul, the soul that makes it alive and gives it its life and power. We draw our vitality and depth from this world soul, anima mundi, one good reason to be in nature, to absorb its soul. This Neoplatonic and transcendentalist outlook offers a deep spiritual motive for staying close to nature, because it is there that we can directly perceive the world's soul and find nourishment for ours.

Another approach is more direct: Find animal Earth by engaging with real animals. Thoreau roused them with his flute, and made sounds with his mouth to summon birds, chipmunks, and fish to keep him company. When hiking with others, he showed them how to avoid harming the plants that were on their path and to be guided by the living creatures around them. He said more than once, how could he be lonely in his small home at Walden Pond with creatures all around him? They are as much persons as we humans are.

Thoreau did not just think all this soul stuff into a theory or a theological rhapsody. He lived it and only then wrote about it. He had the world soul in him, making him into who he became and who he is for us, a channel to the world soul, an offspring of the animal that is Earth, and not a colonizer.

30

FILIBUSTERING TOWARD HEAVEN

The whole enterprise of this nation which is not an upward but a westward one, toward Oregon[,] *California, Japan, &c, is totally devoid of interest to me, whether performed on foot or by a Pacific railroad. It is not illustrated by a thought, it is not warmed by a sentiment, there is nothing in it which one should lay down his life for, nor even his gloves, hardly which one should take up a newspaper for. It is perfectly heathenish—a filibustering toward heaven by the great western route. No, they may go their way to their manifest destiny which I trust is not mine. May my 76 dollars whenever I get them help to carry me in the other direction. I see them on the winding way, but no music "is" wafted from their host, only the rattling of change in their pockets. I would rather be a captive knight, and let them all pass by, than be free only to go whither they are bound. What end do they propose to themselves beyond Japan? What aims more lofty have they than the prairie dogs?*[1]

—Henry David Thoreau to Harrison Gray Otis Blake, February 27, 1853

Manifest Destiny was a belief and an assumption that white settlers in America had a divine right to occupy all land that today is the lower forty-eight states. It promoted slavery and the forcible removal of Native Americans from their land onto reservations. Newspaperman John O'Sullivan used the phrase in 1845, blending a Romantic idea of America's special character with the reality of precious territory expanding westward. It also moved Presidents Andrew Jackson and James K. Polk to be aggressive in taking new territory, including Oregon and Texas.

License to colonize was a hot idea in Henry David Thoreau's time, and he often complained about it. Transforming a slogan about going west into a formula he could live and embody, he said that he did not want to go west, but up. He was interested in the elevation of the human being, not the expansion of its heroic material ambitions. He would like to have heard real music emanating from those rambling trains and coaches, but all he heard was the sound of money.

John Gast's painting of Manifest Destiny, *American Progress* (1872), showing a giant woman leading trains, hikers, and coaches westward, Native Americans cowering at their ominous approach, is still unsettling when the same spirit of entitlement sticks in the American soul. It is the worst form of religious motivation. Painted ten years after Thoreau's death, it is the antithesis of Thoreau's purpose in life and his hope for America.

Up rather than west is a clear graphic for the contrast between Thoreau and many of his countrymen. Today, many enjoy Thoreau the romantic environmentalist, but what about his anticolonialism and his steadfast activity on behalf of abolition? At some risk, he supported John Brown, a prominent and militant abolitionist.

Expanding upward instead of westward included standing boldly for humane values, and Thoreau's journals offer a blueprint for self-discovery, for freely living the life that is natural to you and to you alone. He also moves upward when he advises his reader to select extraordinary literature, to stand on tiptoe when reaching for a book. We would also be following Thoreau's example when listening to music of high value and looking at paintings that are challenging and following only those writers and speakers worthy of attention.

If we take the easy, unaccomplished route, we go westward toward gold that is found in the ground and in our pockets. That is filibustering toward heaven. Going west puts off the truly necessary movement upward. We do something too literal and off-center to avoid the real challenge of elevating our values.

In this sense, many of our actions and decisions, both personal and cultural, distract from the real work of a human being—becoming a noble and perfected person. We are all born for perfection, perfect not as ideal and flawless, but fulfilled, actualized. Yet many of our ambitions aim at outcomes that are neither extraordinary nor noble. In the pursuit of our lives we ourselves are filibustered.

Our whole world of extreme busyness, activity without substantive purpose and achievement, filibusters our need to become more deeply human and to reach high levels of wisdom and understanding. We aim far too low and then spend most of our time traveling west, like the people in *American Progress*, driven emotionally toward the exaggerated and purely financial promise of wealth. Those westward pioneers are going in the wrong direction. Thoreau often said, do not sacrifice lives to acquire Texas, but turn your efforts toward higher goals.

At one time many people entered religious communities to find a life that was thoughtful, values-directed, and aimed at holiness. I did it when I was thirteen years old, spent thirteen years at it, and never regretted that important period in my life. I went up instead of west. During all those years I did not pursue wealth, sex, or a career. My colleagues and I believed we were going after a perfected life of contemplation and intense community.

Money is fine, but you don't have to make it your life purpose. Sex is wonderful, but you don't have to live it compulsively. A career is satisfying, but an increase in knowledge and virtue is ultimately more important. Contributing to humanity is essential.

You may feel that you are a good person because you follow moral teachings you learned as a child. But when you become an adult, you need higher and more subtle ethics. Thoreau did not lie, cheat, or steal, but more significantly, he kept freedom seekers on the Underground Railroad in his own house and accompanied them to Canada. He respected the Native Americans in his part of the world. He promoted serious education for adults in his town. He refused to teach in a school where he was expected to beat his students. He cared for the land, its trees, and its animal inhabitants. He was a failure in love, in publication, and in finance, and he resisted the temptation to filibuster, and yet, gradually, after this death, people all over the world discovered Thoreau as a model of human aspiration.

Thoreau was interested in timing, especially not delaying or postponing action on important values as a way of defeating them. Filibustering is part of life, and we could watch out for it in private life and in public. We get tempted to use delay as a strategy for defeat. Often it can appear to be a good thing, when in fact it is a misleading artifice of avoidance. In many challenging moral situations we may take on the garb of the hero and go west, when the truly challenging way would be to go up.

31

A RESPECTABLE DISTANCE

Let God alone if need be. Methinks, if I loved him more, I should keep him, I should keep myself rather, at a more respectful distance. It is not when I am going to meet him, but when I am just turning away and leaving him alone, that I discover that God is. I say God. I am not sure that that is the name. You will know whom I mean.

—Henry David Thoreau to Harrison
Gray Otis Blake, April 3, 1850

What shall we do with a man who is afraid of the woods, their solitude and darkness? What salvation is there for him? God is silent and mysterious.[1]

—Henry David Thoreau to Harrison
Gray Otis Blake, November 16, 1850

When people ask me if I believe in God, I do not know which the more difficult word is: *God* or *believe*. I have always felt that it is easy to believe in something but more difficult to wrestle with it, to wonder amid doubt and uncertainty. How could you be certain about God?

I appreciate Henry David Thoreau saying that he would keep God at a respectful distance. What a perfect way to describe remaining engaged in the question of God's existence without having an answer or getting too familiar with the God you have uncovered. Wondering about God's existence, rather than assuming it, shows deep respect for a profound, impossible, and perhaps misguided pursuit.

Let God alone. Often, when we talk about whether you believe in God, you are the doer, the active one. But Thoreau, as usual, turns the tables on that assumption. Let God alone. Let God be, whoever and whatever "he" is. Let God take care of God. Most honest religious statements advise us not to interfere. The Tao Te Ching says, "The Tao that can be put into words is not really the Tao." The same could be said about God. The God who can be put into words is not really God. Thomas Aquinas says that we cannot know God in his essence.

When you truly give God a respectful distance, there is not much you can say. And so, Thoreau concludes, "I am not sure that that is the name." Well, no one can be sure, and so the name is provisional. We use it in place of the name we do not know. It may be the only word that is meant to say nothing. You say "God" with the purpose of not saying anything specific, except maybe to say, "God cannot be known or described, so I'll use the name to help me relate to the one I do not know." The name "God" is a placeholder, until you realize that God is not something or someone, and yet is the most important thing of all.

Thoreau lived in a world in which God was a significant player. That is a way of affirming his acknowledgment of God without saying that he believed in God. The transcendentalists sometimes found themselves struggling with language, as when Ralph Waldo Emerson writes that Jesus saw that "God incarnates himself in man, and evermore goes forth anew to take possession of his World."[2] He and Thoreau were both soft mystics who found the divine everywhere.[3]

Thoreau seems to say that if you want to know God, you cannot be afraid of the darkness and solitude of the woods. Maybe he means that relating to the divine is like being in the darkness and yet having a strong sense of where you are. "God is silent and mysterious." This is one of many interesting and innovative thoughts from Thoreau about the sacred in everyday life and in nature. He points to two important aspects of natural religion: a silent divinity and an appreciation for mystery.

Thoreau echoes the ancient tradition of Deus absconditus (the hidden God), that goes back to Isaiah 45:15: "Truly, you are a God who hides himself, O God of Israel, the Savior." The idea was also important to Thomas Aquinas and Martin Luther. For Thoreau, it seems to be another personal and direct discovery from his intimate time with nature. Divinity is there, but you cannot see it.

God has absconded, taken off, gone into hiding, and mystery is the shield that maintains the boundary between the infinite and finite. This is only to say that God is beyond rational explanation and definition. And yet, Thoreau finds him "lurking" in the natural world. If you look closely, you will know that he is there.

These are important passages because Thoreau is aware of divinity in nature and to grasp that understanding is to know him. He is neither an atheist nor a secularist. He comes to nature with a pious attitude, in the sense that he is not a secular scientist, explaining it all through the rules of the scientific method. He seeks out divinity, but his idea of it is not as literal or as dogmatic as most theologians of his time taught. He takes a third path, not necessarily a middle one.

Probably the best source of Thoreau's ideas on natural theology appear in his letters to Harrison Gray Otis Blake, his friend in Worcester, Massachusetts. Happily this correspondence has been compiled into a useful book edited by Bradley P. Dean, *Henry David Thoreau: Letters to a Spiritual Seeker.*

Thoreau's relation to Blake is much like what the Irish call *anam cara*, a soul friend, a solid companionable friendship with the added layer of guidance. Thoreau writes to Blake as if he, Thoreau, were a close friend, and at the same time a valued teacher.

In a letter to Blake from November 20, 1849, Thoreau describes his own spiritual identity. "Depend upon it that rude and careless as I am, I would fain [happily] practise the yoga faithfully." Then he inserts a passage he took from the classic Hindu scripture Mahabharata: "The yogin, absorbed in contemplation, contributes in his degree to creation: he breathes a divine perfume, he hears wonderful things. Divine forms traverse him without tearing him, and united to the nature which is proper to him, he goes, he acts, as animating original matter." He adds, "To some extent and at rare intervals, even I am a yogin."[4]

"He breathes a divine perfume, he hears wonderful things." These are the ways to the divine that Thoreau prized. They are different from what many people demand: intellectual answers and traditional rites and creeds. Typically, Thoreau wanted direct experience, sensual experience, the way he learned nature in his canoe and hiking boots. He went into nature to find divinity lurking there. Apprehending divinity may not be as clear and intellectual as many wish, but Thoreau knew he could find it his own way.

His advice is simple: Let God be. When you leave him alone, that is when you will find him. *Him*, however, is not his preferred pronoun. People insist so desperately that they have the answer about God, as though they have never let him be. Thoreau offers a better model: Do not demand or even expect to know who God is. God is silent and mysterious. That is his nature. Your task is to seek him always and everywhere but also to honor his reticence and keep yourself at a respectable distance.

32

OUR COUSINS THE CATS

Wonderful, wonderful is our life and that of our companions! That there should be such a thing as a brute animal, not human! And that it should attain to a sort of society with our race! Think of cats, for instance. They are neither Chinese nor Tartars. They do not go to school, nor read the Testament; yet how near they come to doing so! How much they are like us who do so! What sort of philosophers are we, who know absolutely nothing of the origin and destiny of cats.[1]

—Henry David Thoreau, journal entry, December 12, 1856

One of the big questions for me that has never been answered is simple: What are animals? With Henry David Thoreau, I wonder about them being so like us and yet so different. They tell me that I am an animal myself, and I see the resemblance, but what are they doing here? How and why do they get along without speech? Why don't they write or express themselves in art?

Once, I was in a lovely bookstore on the East Coast and came across a book of art made by a cat. I bought the book immediately but later was disappointed to find that it was not the art of a real cat but only a joke, as if a cat could create art. My friends thought I was gullible to have been taken in by a spoof, but I had to admit that I would love to see some art works by an animal. It was not difficult for me to accept a cat as an artist and find a book of real cat art.

When I visit my daughter in Ireland I live for a while with her lively, intelligent, and relational dog. Síle is a Mexican Xolo who brings much joy and some annoyance to the household with her exuberance and mischief. Every morning she pounces loudly at our bedroom door and then leaps onto our bed, seconds after my wife and I have wakened, wanting to romp with us and get the day going. When a member of the family has been away for a while, she welcomes this person with lively movements, gestures, and licks, expressing her emotions fully and without any reserve.

Thoreau asks how we can live with a being who doesn't share a common belief or education, and yet we do more than live together. We relate to animals. We form deep bonds and help each other get along and offer companionship and even share what seems to be love. Apparently, what we have in common is sufficient, and that says something about how we relate to other people. Maybe education, a common language, and beliefs don't have to be uniform to make for friendship and joy in being together. Maybe in our relations we should focus more on the animals that we are and develop an animal community among humans. It might be better for us to be together as animals, without our reading and our opinions.

Thoreau observes that cats are neither Chinese nor Tatars. They are not affected by the nations in which they grew up or the language they speak. Yet they know each other in a brief glimpse and respond to each other intensely. We, on the other hand, seem to notice our nationalities first and our humanity second. It's as though we are looking for differences rather than common traits. We want to fight more than we want to cuddle. We don't lick each other unless we know the other really well.

To say that we have much to learn from animals is an understatement. We have everything to learn from them, in part because we are animals, too. Or so it is said. We have so many differences that it is difficult to make such a statement. Rational animals, Thomas Aquinas called us, but that too is a dubious description. We don't act rationally very often. *Homo sapiens* is also a misnomer. Most of the time we are not so sapient.

These statements are much in line with Thoreau's observations about his fellow Concordians. "Though I have been associated even with the select men of this and the surrounding towns, I feel inexpressibly begrimed. My Pegasus has lost his wings; he has turned a reptile and gone on his belly."[2]

My family lived with two dogs during the children's early lives: Little Bear and Luna. Bear was a smart, mischievous, but quiet animal who would often sit with me during psychotherapy sessions. Luna was a beauty and, as her name suggests, a bit otherworldly, and toward the end of her life, rather batty. Bear would sometimes encourage her to get into trouble, but together they gave the family deep joy.

Heartfelt feelings toward animals might lead to other intimacies with the world, like real relationships with trees and hills and fields and stars. You pay close attention to emotions that are not usually at the forefront of daily life. Interest, for example, is sometimes a slight sign of love or joy in seeing one of these things of nature. Knowing that it is love, you can cultivate the relationship and find yourself in world full of cousins. Not just cats and dogs, but plants and rivers and landscapes, as well—cousins all.

A life rich in the friends and relatives of nature is much in the spirit of Thoreau, who never felt alone because of these ever-present relatives. But he was never sentimental about his connections in the world. He lived them as a fact and not a wonder. And this living Earth that he described was not something to imagine for the future, as a distant wish, but a method for being in the world now. It was not New Age but This Age, the world we know and encounter today.

Thoreau was not an easygoing man, but he did not require that others live his lifestyle or adopt his values. He is sometimes called the first environmentalist, but that is not quite right. He did not have the sharp edge of moral persuasion that contemporary environmentalism has. He was strong in his preference to be outdoors and to live close to the land, but the main focus of his work was to discover who he was essentially, to live out as naturally as possible his own potential, and to work out in his writing what it is to be a human being, and in particular, a singular human being.

Thoreau wanted to know how to live with cats in a meaningful way. He probed the connections we have with the natural world and the animal realm. He wanted to penetrate the secrets of a mysterious landscape by living in close relationship with it and probing its habits. He wanted to learn about his own nature as well the nature around him.

"I was going to sit and write or mope all day in the house, but it seems wise to cultivate animal spirits, to embark in enterprises which employ and recreate the whole body," Thoreau writes.[3]

Thoreau, therefore, offers a special definition of environmentalism that includes the self as well as plants and animals. We become who we are potentially through an intimate bond with the natural world. We pursue an ecology of self. We discover what kind of beings we are by observing cats. Our little dog Bear, who would leap two feet in the air, spinning, when he was happy, taught me about pure, unfettered emotion. What he expressed in his vertical leap was love, I am sure: animal love, dog love, an exuberant love that as a human I recognize.

33

EVERY TOWN NEEDS A PARK

Each town should have a park, or rather a primitive forest, of five hundred or a thousand acres, where a stick should never be cut for fuel, a common possession forever, for instruction and recreation. We hear of cow-commons and ministerial lots, but we want men-commons and lay lots, inalienable forever.[1]

—Henry David Thoreau, journal entry, October 15, 1859

Henry David Thoreau lived in a miniature world. Concord, Massachusetts, was the center of the universe, and small Walden Pond was, he often said, the Ganges, the Rivers of Paradise, and the Atlantic Ocean, all in one. Similarly he thought of a park in the heart of a town or city as a primeval forest and a hellish swamp, as the deep muck of its soul. That is to say, the ordinary was extraordinary, both a simple fact of existence and a matter of myth.

An educated imagination allows this kind of worldview, in which you can see the larger picture in the microcosm around you. Thoreau brought this kind of imagination with him wherever he went, and that skill is the basis of his genius. It allowed him to make the leap from the secular to the sacred, and he understood that you can live a full human life only if you can perceive the sacred in the ordinary.

He spent his time in the wilderness of a river, a mountain, or a swamp, and he suggests here that we evoke the wilderness in a town park, which we should make as wild as possible within the limits of the civilized space. A deep mystery lies behind this calculation. Pars pro toto. Part for the whole. A miniature forest in the middle of a town has the power to make the spirit of a wilder wilderness accessible to the townspeople. You need the spirit of that wilderness to complete the contoured world in which you live. You are trying to create an imaginal wild, not a literal one, and you can invoke that spirit with a park, suitably untamed and rich in diversity.

Human beings can transmute the local into the universal, and the personal into the archetypal. The great twentieth-century scholar of myth and religion Mircea Eliade writes: "What is essential in mythical behavior—the exemplary pattern, the repetition, the break with profane duration and integration into primordial time."[2] To Eliade, primordial time happens before time begins or is equivalent to the timeless. He goes on by relating this pattern to the shift in personalities from historical to mythic. "A very general human tendency; namely, to hold up one life-history as a paradigm and turn the historical personage into an archetype."[3] We can do the same with a piece of land, transform it from a literal park to a mythic, fantasy wilderness.

Thoreau had this idea ingrained in him and habitually thought in this mythmaking way. Walden Pond is the Ganges River and the woods around it the Garden of Eden. When he recommends a primeval park in every town, he is not just asking for space in which to refresh yourself bodily. He wants a return to Eden or to the sacred renewal of the Ganges. He hopes that in a park the citizen will find a fantasy of wilderness and not only its physical elements. That is why it should be big and pristine. It must produce an effect on the soul and spirit and not just serve as recreation. It takes a push to move from literal refreshment to the enchantment of myth. This could be an important principle in restoring humanity to our world: To know how to touch the hearts of people with these profound and life-enhancing creations, how to make myth out of the ordinary stuff of life.

When Thoreau says that a stick should never be cut for fuel, he is speaking the way a caretaker of the sacred speaks. It takes only a single infraction to ruin the unbroken temenos, the borders of a sacred space. At Christmas, it takes someone only to say, "There is no Santa Claus," to break the spell. One way this sacralization is accomplished in India, Japan, and other traditional places is to use rituals in the making of the space or following traditional methods of construction and the careful use of images. You could also take care not to take things literally or secularly too often. Slight excursions from the mythos of a place, such as using it for practical purposes, destroys the halo of holiness that keeps it sacred.

When people create a public space today, the most thoughtful of them use their intuition and artistic sense to be effective and to offer something of value to the public, but in Western countries they may lack the guidance of tradition with all its wisdom, method, and skill. They may especially lack the power to evoke archetypal figures and settings. Thoreau offers a simple suggestion for preserving the sanctity of the town park: Do not cut any sticks for fuel. In other words, do not turn the sacred space into a practical resource. This small infraction could break the spell.

In Thoreau's time, special spaces were reserved for cows and for ministers. He suggests instead "men-commons" and "lay lots." Reserve space for people who are not ministers. At a deeper level, this might mean leaving behind purely practical concerns, like providing pasture for cows. Make it a people commons. And do not just respect religious ministers, but laypeople, too. Bring the sacred into our secular world and thereby infuse the secular with sacred themes.

A raw park in a town may conceal an opening to divinity, because people will generally treat it in secular terms by not giving it enough spiritual attention or seeing it as a place mainly for physical exercise. Certain forms in nature, such as cone-shaped mountains and deep wells and certain caves and grottoes, evoke a natural piety and reverence. A simple town park, full of nature's spirituality, might also grace a city with a special spirit that offers the community an ordinary source of reverence and contemplation.

The challenge will be to keep the park pristine and not overdeveloped or overused. It will require steady care and attention so that the holiness is not lost to development and exploitation. In my ideal world we would have professional natural theologians whose job it would be to prevent the oversecularization of culture.

A park is not just for the body, but also for the soul. It can help relieve anxiety by keeping us in touch with natural forms and processes, leading us back to our original natures and connecting us to the eternal elements of trees and rocks and streams, touching the bedrock of a self. Without a park we live our daily lives in shallow secular ground, especially in modern times when we have lost touch with deep natural designs and processes. We need parks, built and sustained in an atmosphere of the holy, to maintain our humanity.

Frederick Law Olmsted—the famous landscape architect who designed New York's Central Park, Montreal's Mount Royal, Stanford

University, the US Capitol grounds, and other special spaces—developed a sophisticated philosophy of parks. Their natural components, he said, can offer healing and restorative forces to citizens and have a civilizing effect. Just being in a good park you can acquire these benefits. No one has to explain a park to you or give you a page of instructions. Much larger national parks and reserves serve a similar purpose and therefore are necessary and precious.

In this Thoreau was a forerunner, because he always said that nature can heal and civilize, and even a relatively small park, carefully crafted, can have these effects. To live the Thoreau philosophy you do not have to be a farmer or live in a small town. You can tend a special plant in your home, miniaturizing the wilderness like a bonsai tree, creating a separate reality, a slice of myth, that can make life worth living.

34

MY OWN SACRAMENTS

I find that I conciliate the gods by some sacrament as bathing, or abstemiousness in diet, or rising early, and directly they smile on me. These are my sacraments. Why should we be related as mortals merely, as limited to one state of existence? Our lives are immortal, our transmigrations are infinite . . . I would meet my friend not in the light or shadow of our human life alone—but as daimons. We should not be less tender and human sympathizing for this because we should meet intimately as essences . . . The undertaker will have a dusty time that undertakes to bury me. I go with the party of the gods . . . They are benighted, they are ineffectual men who walk in the valley of the shadow of Death. I am not a-going to be a man merely, I will be Hari.[1]

—Henry David Thoreau,
journal entry, July 30, 1848

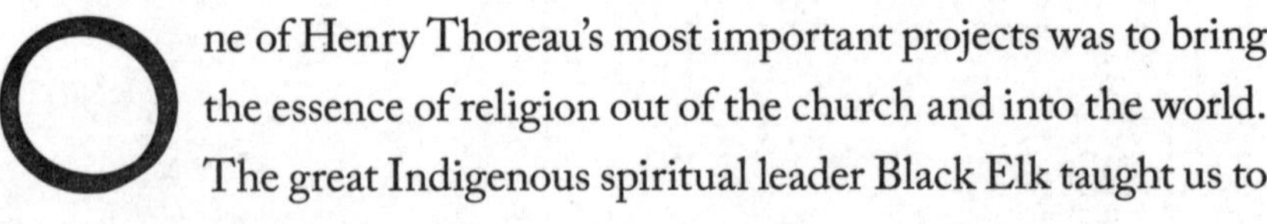

One of Henry Thoreau's most important projects was to bring the essence of religion out of the church and into the world. The great Indigenous spiritual leader Black Elk taught us to see "in a sacred manner." Thoreau developed that capacity in his own way as consistently throughout his life he looked at the things around him—including animals, swamps, and rivers—and beheld the sacred. He saw salvation in a perch swimming in Walden Pond and a holy ritual in going for a daily walk. For him, getting up early, restricting his eating, and going for a swim were sacraments, which have been defined as "outward forms of an inward grace." These actions also happen to be central activities in a monk's daily life, and Thoreau became a new kind of monk, one whose life of holy perfection was natural and profoundly secular and vernacular.

Thoreau's sacraments transformed the quotidian into the spiritual and the ordinary secular into the monastic. His approach to simple life habits helped redefine monastic life so that even today it might be lived outside any actual monastery. This transformation of formal religion into ordinary, secular spiritual practice could be one of the most significant achievements of our time, although it probably will not happen seriously until we have a new visionary generation, one that can transcend the rigid formalism of highly structured religion.

Religions often recommend fasting, immersion in water, and early rising as part of a monastic routine—as a former monk I speak from experience. Thoreau does not use the word, but he "borrows" certain rituals from traditional religion so that they become sacraments in his own way of life.

He adapts another rich idea from the ancient Greek tradition, where classic writings speak of a daimon, an invisible power, something like an angel, that can warn, inspire, and sometimes compel a person. Plato's Socrates celebrated his daimon, which warned him against doing the wrong things; William Butler Yeats described his daimon as a presence that cooperated in making his life and poetry; Carl Jung named his guiding daimon Philemon; James Hillman spoke of the daimon as an essential guardian; Simone Weil speaks of the daimon as an "invisible friend"; and Elizabeth Bishop as "Man-moth." In Anne Carson's vivid translation of Euripides's *Bakkhai*, the god Dionysus says: "I am something supernatural, not exactly god, ghost, spirit, angel, principle or element—there is no term for it in English. In Greek they say daimon."[2] Carson nails this mysterious word exactly by saying what it is not.

We should encounter our friends not just as regular human beings and not as gods, but as members of an "invisible friendship," an other-than-human and yet not too far out in the stratosphere being who nevertheless does not give up human tenderness. There is more to us than can be explained by our earthiness and ordinariness. We have a powerful and defining essence that cannot be seen but can be detected as a force in our presentation of ourselves and in our relationships.

Thinking of his daimon, Thoreau asserts that he is not in life to be a mere human, but to be Hari, or Vishnu, the Indian god who banishes illusion. You can discern daimonic people by the force of their character and by noticing how they live by inspiration. Thoreau served and even embodied Vishnu in the passion that set him afire in his deliberate and creative life and in how he did everything he could to lift the veil of illusion, which in his case meant discovering how to live and what to write.

When the guiding forces of life are with us, we are more than human. Therefore, in community, we are an odd assembly. If we could picture the greater scene, we would see us gathered together with our daimons, ourselves accompanied by or empowered by more-than-human, yet still natural, forces and powers. Thoreau's idea of the daimon echoes the famous lines of another inspired figure who found spiritual significance in the natural world, Pierre Teilhard de Chardin: "We are not human beings having a spiritual experience. We are spiritual beings having a human experience."

We can stop talking about ourselves as a human race. We are more than human, possessed by an indwelling and outdwelling spirit. The outer one, especially for Thoreau, is not only a town having inspired human beings but the fertile swamps that surround that town. There you can meet the daimon, because nature is the habitat of spirits and powers beyond human scope. According to Thoreau, you will find them in the swampy ravines even more so than on the mountaintops and certainly more so than on the streets or in buildings. Why else climb uplifting mountains or explore muddy terrain than to encounter the powers, the daimons, that dwell there?

If you are enlivened by the daimon, you will not feel constantly threatened by the inevitability of death. You live this life as a preparation for a different life, maybe the fulfillment of the essence that is active in mortal years but has a more extended potentiality. The green life. The life of plants and trees and flowers, each moving through their respective seasons, eternally, year after year, perennials rooted in timelessness.

Thoreau could live in his unique way and write in his mind-bending style because he was close to his daimonic nature. He followed its promptings, even in such a small thing as going for a walk without making plans, letting the daimon choose the way. That small daily ritual, as well as his encounters with fish, fed his natural spirituality.

Could this be our problem in the twenty-first century—that we have not yet discovered that we are more than human? Is that why so many are fascinated with UFOs and science fiction? Are we trying to survive with our mere biological selves, forgetting, as the old tales show, that we are more than that, that we are daimonic creatures, half-human and half-angel, ourselves visitors from outer space? We, too, are aliens living on a planet in a vast cosmos possessed of preternatural powers, provided we allow them to empower us.

The visionary theologian of the fifteenth century, Nicholas of Cusa, defined the human being as *deus humanus*, a human god. Although philosophy in the European Renaissance gave rise to a new humanism, it did so by building on the idea that human beings are more than biological beings. We are human because of the divinity that can reside in us. Similarly, Thoreau stated that humans are not biologically defined but have an otherworldly component, that the angel, the daimon, and divinity itself are factors in our existence.

35

MY INNER EASTWARD MOUNTAIN

If you have been to the top of Mount Washington, let me ask, what did you find there? That is the way they prove witnesses, you know. Going up there and being blown on is nothing. We never do much climbing while we are there, but we eat our luncheon, etc., very much as at home. It is after we get home that we really go over the mountain, if ever. What did the mountain say: What did the mountain do?[1]

—Henry David Thoreau to Harrison Gray Otis Blake, November 16, 1857

I keep a mountain anchored off eastward a little way, which I ascend in my dreams both awake and asleep. Its broad base spreads over a village or two, which do not know it; neither does it know them, nor do I when I ascend it. I can see its general outline as plainly now in my mind as that of Wachusett. I do not invent in the least but state exactly what I see. I find that

I go up it when I am light-footed and earnest. It ever smokes like an altar with its sacrifice. I am not aware that a single villager frequents it or knows of it. I keep this mountain to ride instead of a horse.[2]

—Henry David Thoreau, journal entry, November 12, 1859

I do not know how to distinguish between our waking life and a dream. Are we not always living the life that we imagine we are?[3]

—Henry David Thoreau, journal entry, May 27, 1841

What is the best way to climb a mountain? The climb itself is not the main thing, especially not the actual sights and sensations of being high and in the wind. The truly significant thing is the mountain you remember and that stays in your fantasy. Did the mountain speak to you? Was anything about it unexpected? How do you hold it in you now that the climb is over? Will it play a role in your future life?

You climb a mountain to have it with you forever, giving you its lessons, even taking you to new places as if it were a vehicle for your mind and heart. Henry David Thoreau anticipates psychologies of the imagination that only today are allowing us to sense the reality status of the imagined. Here he describes living intensely in an imaginal world. Not imaginary—one that is not real or is an escape—but an imaginal realm, where fantasy and reality overlap to create a real presence. Thoreau's "mountain anchored off eastward," a purely imaginal one, served him better than a physical one.

But you find Thoreau living in these dual realms continuously, as when he considers that Walden Pond was there in the Garden of Eden. His imagination expands his world significantly, allowing him to glide from this time and place to the era and geography of elsewhere. His eastward mountain stretches over villages, but the people there do not know of it. They live in a different landscape where the imagination is not real. Like most of us, they are in clock time and map space. On the other hand, Thoreau is a natural mystic and lives partly in time and partly in the timeless, as the Renaissance philosopher Marsilio Ficino said of the soul.

In this way Thoreau has a shamanic aspect, since he can traverse worlds by moving deftly from the actual to the imaginal. Like the mythic shamans, Pan and Orpheus, he turns to music, especially his flute, to cross the borders. Interestingly, Thoreau uses the term *tintinnabulum* for his music, the word the contemporary spiritual composer Arvo Pärt uses for the simple musical structures he uses to create his otherworldly sounds.

In these ways Thoreau connects with *magia naturalis* (natural magic) as practiced by Ficino and his followers over the ages. This is music not so much for aesthetic purposes as for spiritual and psychological benefits. With his flute, Thoreau lures animals out of their dens and calms people at a funeral. He mentions a dream that reveals how essential music was to him: "The instant I awoke, methought I was a musical instrument from which I heard a strain die out,—a bugle, or a clarionet, or a flute. My body was the organ and channel of melody, as a flute is of the music that is breathed through it. My flesh sounded and vibrated still to the strain, and my nerves were the chords of the lyre."[4]

This dream might give a hint as to how connected Thoreau was to the world around him. In the dream, he was not just playing the flute but was the flute. His body, he writes, vibrated with the sound and his nerves were like the shimmering, sounding strings. When we try to learn from him how to be a natural person, we might imagine being so intensely engaged with the world. We do not play our experience of the world on an instrument, we are the instrument. We do not merely record our experience of nature, we are it.

A flute emits beautiful sounds as the player's breath flows through the long pipe, and the lengths of the flow are changed as fingers stop holes in the body of the instrument. The flute extends the breath of the player and changes the quality of its sound. Its body and the player's body together go out into the world, manifesting beauty.

In his dream Thoreau was making music without any separation between him and his instrument. He was the instrument. When he climbed a mountain, the mountain shape-shifted into an imaginal mountain and was established in him. It became impossible to distinguish him from his world or his fantasies about it.

The "mountain anchored off eastward" is a remarkable example of this process of shifting from actual to imaginal. Thoreau's neighbors would never see his eastern mountain, yet for him it was a source of confidence. Similarly, for him, playing the flute was being the flute. "I do not know how to distinguish between our waking life and a dream."

I sit with clients in therapy and try to hear the eastern mountains and magical flutes in their lives and histories. This is where meaning lies hidden and, revealed, tells of the themes that cause pain or that offer a strong identity. The Shakers in Thoreau's time referred to their members who were especially tuned in to inspiration as "instruments." In our day we need "instruments," too, people who can receive inspiration from that otherworld that Thoreau knew so well. We ourselves could be instruments, able to receive the hidden mysteries of the world for our daily benefit.

The modern way is to make little of the imaginal and even see it as insane, but to hear Thoreau's teaching, we could take the bold step into fantasy, learn its rules, and be elevated by it. We could become flutes and guitars and pianos and even hold a special eastern mountain in our imaginations. If that suggestion seems extreme, then maybe we should learn from Thoreau to push the limits and be imaginative people in the most radical ways.

36

THE PHILOSOPHY OF WOOD

I do not know how to distinguish between our waking life and a dream. Are we not always living the life that we imagine we are?

Philosophy is a Greek word by good rights, and it stands almost for a Greek thing. Yet some rumor of it has reached the commonest mind. Martial Miles, who came to collect his wood bill to-day, said, when I objected to the small size of his wood, that it was necessary to split wood fine in order to cure it well, that he had found that wood that was more than four inches in diameter would not dry, and moreover a good deal depended on the manner in which it was corded up in the woods. He piled his high and tightly. If this were not well done the stakes would spread and the wood lie loosely, and so the rain and snow find their way into it. And he added, "I have handled a good deal of wood, and I think that I understand the philosophy of it."[1]

—Henry David Thoreau, *Walden*

The word *philosophy* comes from two Greek words, *philo* and *Sophia. Philo* means "love." I capitalized Sophia because in ancient times she was a female quasi-divine spirit closely associated with God, if not the female manifestation of God. Later she became the personification of wisdom and later still the simple idea of wisdom. Therefore, *philosophy*, from its etymology and from mythology, means "the love of wisdom," and has a noble history.

Wisdom is not the same as knowledge. Deeper and somewhat more practical, it is an intelligence needed to live a good life, attained after a long apprenticeship or search. A rocket scientist may be intelligent but not necessarily wise. Wisdom is set deep in the heart, giving blood and vitality to the dry ideas stored in the mind.

Henry David Thoreau's homely account would take us further into the meaning of wisdom and therefore of philosophy. In an academic setting philosophy may be rational and abstract, treating subtle definitions and faint points of language. Sometimes it is more concrete and personal. Albert Camus's novels are considered philosophy, as is Robert M. Persig's *The Zen of Motorcycle Maintenance*, with its highly personal exploration of the meaning and experience of quality.

Many philosophers discuss the nature of things, and the *philo* element is often present and palpable. Philosophers love their penetrating explorations of an idea. Sophia as wisdom is more often absent, as discussions become airy and thin in the ionosphere of rare thought and lofty abstraction. Thoreau's story shows a lowering of the very idea of philosophy. When you begin discussing the philosophy of wood, you have brought thought down to earth.

Not all philosophers are abstract. One I studied in my teens, Gabriel Marcel, known as a Catholic existentialist, wrote plays and probing, episodic essays. He was famous for exploring the difference between a problem and a mystery, an issue that appealed to me in my early college years. Thomas Aquinas used strict syllogisms and logic to explore the entire universe, while Marcel examined human experience, especially the ways people respond to tragedy and how they form bonds.

I have an odd story about Marcel that echoes Thoreau's tale about wood. I was studying in Northern Ireland and often traveled to Dublin, where one day I had an appointment to visit Thomas McGreevy, director of the National Gallery of Ireland. I was nineteen. I had become frustrated with the cold logic of classical philosophy and, in search of a more humanistic approach, began reading Marcel.

I arrived at the main office of the director at the gallery in time to see a small, dark-haired man rushing out. When I saw McGreevy, who had become my friend, I asked him who that out-of-control man was. "Oh, that was Gabriel Marcel, the existentialist, you know, just here for a quick visit." I was sorry I hadn't run into him and shared a cup of tea with him, but it wasn't to be. At least I had a brush, literally, with a philosopher who was not abstract.

When I began practicing psychotherapy and friends heard how I was doing it, they would tease me by saying that I was a practical philosopher and that people were coming to me for philosophical advice. I didn't mind the label at all, because I do think that what we call psychological issues are often matters of theology and philosophy. I also recommend to people that they each come up with their own philosophy of life, and I like to take advantage of some public occasions where I can say that I am a theologian, which, to me, is a philosopher interested in gods, angels, and mysteries.

If everyone took a vivid interest in the love of wisdom, we would be a more thoughtful people. Philosophy need not be lofty or dry and intellectual. It begins in wonder and moves on to a close examination of whatever captures your heart. It is a *love* of wisdom, not only an intellectual pursuit of it.

You can be philosophical about anything and everything, meaning that you can consider the most ordinary things in the context of everything and wonder what they mean and where they fit. How do they fulfill themselves and what do they offer? I like to philosophize about art, its place in life, and its makers.

Martial Miles stopped at Thoreau's house one day to be paid for some logs he had delivered. He told Thoreau why he cut the logs short and narrow and then explained that over the years he had come to know the philosophy of wood. He had become wise about wood, and that wisdom led to his practical skill at sizing logs properly and ultimately helping Thoreau stay warm in the New England winter. Philosophy can offer comfort.

I recall that once, early in my career, I was asked to give a lecture at a booksellers' convention. It was held at a massive convention center in a big city. I was told that some in attendance were publishers' representatives and that some of them were thinking of leaving the profession. I gave them a lecture about the book: its early history, etymologies, the way the book evolved over centuries, and what a beautiful and important thing it is. A philosophy of the book. Afterward, a few reps came up to me and told me they had been thinking of quitting their jobs but I had inspired them to remain in publishing. I felt that the return of love for books was accomplished by philosophy.

It would not hurt to philosophize about every little thing in our lives. We do not think deeply enough about the things around us, and so we do not love them. It takes little effort to become a mundane, practical philosopher, a lover of wisdom. Its practice could bring us closer to our world, one of Thoreau's primary aims in life.

37

THE MOUTH OF A REPTILE

There is a reptile in the throat of a greedy man always thirsting and famishing. It is not his own natural hunger and thirst which he satisfies . . . Is there not such a thing as getting rid of the snake which you have swallowed when young, when thoughtless you stooped and drank at stagnant waters, which has worried you in your waking hours and in your sleep ever since, and appropriated the life that was yours?[1]

—Henry David Thoreau, journal entry, September 2, 1851

Better for me, says my genius, to go cranberrying this afternoon, than go consul for Liverpool . . . and get I don't know how many thousand dollars for it, with no such flavor . . . Let not your life be wholly without an object, though it be only to ascertain the flavor of a cranberry, for it will not be only the quality of an insignificant berry that you will have tasted, but the flavor of your life to that extent, and it will be such a sauce as no wealth can buy.[2]

—Henry David Thoreau, journal entry, August 30, 1856

O how I laugh when I think of my vague indefinite riches. No run on my bank can drain it—for my wealth is not possession but enjoyment.[3]

—Henry David Thoreau to Harrison Otis Blake, December 6, 1856

When I was a monk living under a vow of poverty, I was given many reasons for the vow, but never heard Henry David Thoreau's idea that doing without is something to be enjoyed and pursued as a good thing. Not only does it give you a challenge, not having what other people feel is necessary or even what you think you need, it enriches life. For one thing, it steers you toward "possessions" that offer deep and lasting pleasure. Thoreau would say that you realize that you have sunsets, the fresh aroma of trees, and the tang of berries. Nothing you could buy could give you such deep satisfaction.

The spirit of poverty, meaning nonownership, naturally gives birth to an appreciation for the commons, for the fresh air and inspiring landscape and naturally growing food. The commons includes the natural world available to us all. Some refer to it as "borrowed" property, like the mile-long pond where I live with my wife in view of Mount Monadnock, which is also borrowed and part of the commons. Thoreau would say that the pond and the mountain make us wealthy even though we do not own any of it.

Thoreau explains that ruinous greed is not the fault of any person but of a strong reptile presence down in a person's gut, a snake that accounts for an unsatisfied hunger for things. This snake is not a simple metaphor but perhaps close to Sigmund Freud's sexual theory of orality, seeing greed as an unconscious desire related to an infant's need for oral stimulation in sucking and eating. Thoreau's snake is an abdominal mouth wanting not only food but, by extension, many kinds of satisfactions, like money and possessions.

At some time in your past, you must have inadvertently swallowed a snake whose open mouth still gives you cravings. As an adult you can feel it there, especially in your inability to be sated—with money, possessions, sex, experiences. A feral hunger keeps your desire for possessions focused on the things that you imagine will save you from the pale lethargy of everyday existence. You go after almost any object that cannot satisfy your craving but can point to what you lack. This swallowed, ever-present internal oral compulsion accounts for an uncontrollable lust for things, especially things you do not need.

It is normal to desire things and to enjoy possessions. Purchasing can bring joy and even have a therapeutic effect. But greed is desire that has become a psychological disorder, a problem in which normal hunger is now out of control. To deal with it, you could imagine something foreign inside you that has taken over and is difficult to resist. You can ask yourself, where did I pick up this strong longing to possess?

To deal with the obsession you can transform your hunger for things into feasting on the natural world, enjoying plants, trees, and animals in their own settings rather than possessing them. You do not need to snatch things from their environment and bring them into your own space, as if you were swallowing them, but you can take pleasure in them at a distance. Let things be free and resist the temptation to incorporate them into your domain. Thoreau's standard substitute for possessing things is to enjoy picking berries and eating them in the wild.

The trouble with greed is that it tends to take over and leave no room for other worthwhile values. When people assume that having more money and a bigger house and infinite possessions will bring happiness, these preoccupations make it difficult to be generous to those who have little. Having too many possessions also stands in the way of finding pleasure in what you do not possess. In this way greed is one of the major blocks to a happy life and a healthy society.

In addition, greed promotes an egotistical psychology, an emphasis on *me* rather than *we*. You may think you are better because you own more than most. You are in the one percent. For a healthy society we need a deep community feeling to ground a cooperative citizenry. You may be thinking, Thoreau did not have much community feeling. True, he did not have much faith in a materialistic culture, and he based his life of community in his direct and intimate relations with the natural world, but he also participated in the justice and educational aspects of his hometown of Concord. In all of this he models a way of life that is in the spirit of the commons and the deep practice of democracy.

How can we enjoy the beauty of the world when we strive to keep it all hoarded in our homes? One way is to go with the symptom instead of making it a curse. Maybe the strength of our greed is a good thing. It can be beneficial to have a powerful lust for life. Greedy people may have to work hard to obtain the large sums of money necessary for all their properties. They expect praise for their ambition and effort. But the object of their desire may be misplaced. Thoreau sometimes says that others take pleasure in fine houses and property, while he has the huge enjoyment of the rivers on which he boats and the mountains he climbs. In that way he is rich beyond measure. His "wealth" lies in his extraordinary participation in the natural world. An appetite for life is not the problem, but collecting objects may not fulfill that appetite. The problem is not a hunger for riches but a faulty idea of what kind of wealth you want.

As you watch many sunsets and swim in beautiful bodies of water you find that there is a natural and common kind of property. You do not need a huge bank account for it. Instead of craving many commonly valued objects, such as the very latest in technology or things that make life merely convenient, you could discover the joy of planting flowers and vegetables or discovering a luscious view of nature or cooking unusual dishes from around the world. This is greed of a different sort, and it is a strategy that Thoreau employed for himself. He was greedy for closer contact with life.

In his essay on Medusa, the petrifying, ugly monster who had snakes for hair, Freud said that the many snakes signify castration. In that way, the display of many possessions shows that, deep down, you have nothing. Owning too many things may indicate that you do not have the joy of owning any of them. It would be better to have one thing that truly brings you joy than to have many that have little meaning or are so transitory that they fail to touch your heart.

In a society lacking soul, people may assume that the purpose of life is to have a luxurious lifestyle, or as close to it as you can get. They are impressed by celebrity and the display of wealth, and the images of greed and high living that afflict us daily make the snake hungrier. You approach life with your mouth, with an oral need for satisfaction. A different oral satisfaction might be to kiss the world and establish an erotic connection to it rather than a consuming one.

When I am in Ireland or England, in the country or in small towns, I enjoy seeing the sheep grazing on the green hills just outside of the city. I don't own these sheep, but they give me more joy and pleasure than other fancy things I could own. Sometimes I think that the reason I travel to Ireland, England, and Scotland is to stand in a town and watch the sheep up on the hills. I feel a sudden surge of true wealth, and I am temporarily released from the greed that does not offer such pleasures. I become wealthy in the things that matter and that touch the heart.

38

THE POETRY OF FISH

I cannot but see still in my mind's eye those little striped breams poised in Walden's glaucous water . . . the miracle of its existence, my contemporary and neighbor, yet so different from me! I can only poise my thought there by its side and try to think like a bream for a moment. I can only think of precious jewels, of music, poetry, beauty, and the mystery of life. I only see the bream in its orbit, as I see a star, but I care not to measure its distance or weight. The bream, appreciated, floats in the pond as the centre of the system, another image of God . . . It is as if a poet or an anchorite had moved into the town, whom I can see from time to time and think of yet oftener . . . One boy thinks of fishes and goes a-fishing from the same motive as his brother searches the poets for rare lines. It is the poetry of fishes which is their chief use. The beauty of the fish, that is what is best worth the while to measure. Its place in our systems is of comparatively little importance. Generally the boy loses some of his perception and his interest in the fish; he degenerates into a fisherman or an ichthyologist.[1]

—Henry David Thoreau, journal entry, November 30, 1858

Henry David Thoreau often refers to fish he encounters, and often he elevates the fish to high levels of meaning. Here a fish in the pond evokes beauty and the mystery of life. An image of God, no less. One thinks of the image of the fish in Christianity, but, of course, Thoreau is thinking of natural religion, not a belief system, religion rooted in a poetic sensibility, that can see divinity in every element of nature, including fish.

Jesus told his followers to stop fishing for fish and fish for humans. In that spirit Thoreau employs a broader meaning, not only to fishing but also to fish. He refers to a person fishing for good lines in poems. He sees the bream swimming in the lake as the center of the system, the solar system, and an image of God himself.

Fish live in their own domain, in a body of water, and are generally invisible. I live on a lake that is full of fish, but I don't see even one often. In that regard, Thoreau associates the fish to an anchorite, a monk or holy person who withdraws from society for spiritual reasons. This is another example of fish poetry. The fish as a hermit or a cloistered monk, or the monk as a fish.

Being near a body of water you are in the mysterious area where a whole social life is going on invisibly close by. The mystery can be haunting, and it may remind you that the whole world is like that. Lives are being lived under water, deep in the earth, in the sky. What is our plane of existence, and how does it define who we are?

Edward O. Wilson, who focused his attention on ants, says about a sight he came upon in Brazil: "The first worker ants came scurrying purposefully out of the surrounding forest. They were brick-red in color, about a quarter-inch in length, and bristling with short, sharp spines. Within minutes several hundred had arrived . . . Within an hour the trickle expanded to twin rivers of tens of thousands of ants running ten or more abreast."[2]

Psychoanalysts have used the image of the ocean for the unconscious level of human life. Carl Jung writes about the unconscious as filled with "stars, sparks and luminous fish eyes."[3] In fact, Jung wrote an entire book, *Aion*, on the image of the fish, where he mentions that in Jewish tradition devout Israelites who live in the water of the doctrine are likened to fishes. Along those lines, you could say that we are all fish swimming in the deep waters of culture.

The fish, then, is a good basis for metaphorical extravagance. I doubt that I could ever end poetizing the fish. But Thoreau anchors his metaphors in the actual fish that he sees in the pond. He does not lose the fish for the fish images. He remains in the dialogue of actual fish and fish metaphors. He keeps paddling on the Assabet River, and daily he scans Walden Pond for the fish that feed his imagination. Here is yet another principle of imagination: Find nature's potent metaphors, but never give up contemplating nature's actual wonders.

At the end of his far-reaching rhapsody on fish, Thoreau remarks about how a young person might lose his appreciation of the metaphor of fish, and instead become a fisherman or an ichthyologist, two ways to lose track of the necessary metaphor. Finally, he says that a fish is an image of God. He moves from imagination to natural religion. You start with a special sight, the bream in the pond. This mysterious alien in the pond places you in a state of wonder, possibly even a small trance, as you concentrate on the nature of fish. Then you wonder about all creatures living their lives in their own universes. You begin to understand that life itself is mysterious. You wonder what it is all about. You wonder if God is at work, and if it is so, if the fish a manifestation of God.

You do not need a belief in God to have this experience. Just let the word *God* stand for the mystery of it all. Allow the mystery to be perceived by wonder rather than belief. Or do not use the word *God* at all, if that is better for you. Do not worry about belief and nonbelief, as so many do. Relax with the enchantment of it all and allow Thoreau to illuminate and educate your imagination. The main point about fish is their poetry, how they point beyond themselves to the ultimate mysteries and beauties.

Thoreau hints that the poetics and the beauty of a fish go together. You can see this interchange in a painting. If the image does not point beyond itself to a deeper and more meaningful level, then its beauty is diminished. If you do not see the poetry of a fish, you may admire its form and color, but the fish as an evocative and stirring image may be lost. It would be like looking at a serious painting, noting the subject matter and form, but overlooking layers of meaning.

In this passage we also see Thoreau's brand of transcendentalism. It isn't just nature that he calls on for a remarkable life, but this individual fish that is like a star in the sky and at the same time is his "contemporary and neighbor." We are all in this human life with certain coordinates of time and space. It is significant to Thoreau that the fish he sees in the pond shares these coordinates and therefore has a special intimate relationship with Thoreau.

The fish circling in the pond is as mysterious and significant as a planet orbiting the sun. We keep an eye on these beings so that we know who we are and how to make sense of our lives. It all has to do with the poetry of fish, whether they are orbiting your pond and lake or swimming in your unconscious imagination. You can find them in the pool of your soul, playing a part in your experience of life.

39

ROOM FOR THOUGHT

One inconvenience I sometimes experienced in so small a house, the difficulty of getting to a sufficient distance from my guest when we began to utter the big thoughts in big words. You want room for your thoughts to get into sailing trim and run a course or two before they make their port. The bullet of your thought must have overcome its lateral and ricochet motion and fallen into its last and steady course before it reaches the ear of the hearer, else it may plough out again through the side of his head. Also, our sentences wanted room to un-fold and form their columns in the interval. Individuals, like nations, must have suitable broad and natural boundaries, even a considerable neutral ground, between them. I have found it a singular luxury to talk across the pond to a companion on the opposite side. In my house we were so near that we could not begin to hear,—we could not speak low enough to be heard; as when you throw two stones into calm water so near that they break each other's undulations. If we are merely loquacious and loud talkers, then we can afford to stand very near together, cheek by jowl, and feel each other's breath; but if we speak reservedly and thoughtfully, we want to be farther apart, that all animal heat and moisture may have a chance to evaporate. If we would enjoy the most intimate society with that in each of us which is without, or above, being spoken to, we must not only be silent, but commonly so far apart bodily that we cannot possibly hear each other's voice in any case. Referred to this standard, speech is for the convenience of those who are hard of hearing; but there are many fine things which we cannot say if we have to shout. As the conversation began to assume a loftier and grander tone, we gradually shoved our chairs farther apart till they touched the wall in opposite corners, and then commonly there was not room enough.[1]

—Henry David Thoreau, *Walden*

This entry, full of "tall stories" of trying to find a big enough space for a thoughtful conversation, reveals Henry David Thoreau's humor and his thick metaphorical way of making a good point. Ideas are big and weighty. Elsewhere he writes that you should stand on your tiptoes to read the best and most lofty books, and here he adds that you need enough space for your expansive thoughts.

It makes a difference how much space you have around you and between you in a significant interchange. I recall a conversation I had with Huston Smith, the highly respected religion scholar, on a bus en route to a conference, sitting next to each other with hardly any space between us. It was not only uncomfortable but awkward trying to talk with our heads so close to each other. Truly, there was no room for a good idea.

On the other hand, I also remember a conversation I had in an empty hotel ballroom, after presenting a lecture with Pat Toomay, my writer friend who played professional football for the Dallas Cowboys. The room was just too big and empty for Pat and me to explore the complex ideas that kept coming up, and we had to seek a smaller space. A tight nook near a bar and news shop helped the conversation flow and focus.

Thoreau says that in his 10 x 15 foot house he and his friends could not speak low enough to be heard. Maybe the figure of speech here is a form of antiphrasis, using words in a sense opposite to their meaning, possibly it is simply irony. It would be equivalent to saying, "Speak more softly, please. I can't hear what you are saying." Our selection is an extended wordplay in which you say the opposite of what you intend to make your point with exaggeration and wit.

One somewhat less literal point Thoreau makes is that living in a small house, like the one he built at Walden Pond, has its drawbacks. It's true of everyone: You must adjust to the scope of your space, where you live or where you find yourself, not only for conversations but for living in general.

I have always preferred a large house. When we came into some money, a rare occasion, my wife and I once had a large house built, and I enjoyed it. This house had a walk-in pantry and a small suite for a live-in au pair. My wife says that for me this taste for a large living space is a carryover from spending my teens and twenties living in monasteries, which tended to be grand.

Thoreau's topsy-turvy reasoning about space and conversation was deeply rooted. Many people refer to his home at Walden Pond as a cabin. Visit the replica cabin at Walden today, and you will understand. But he always spoke of it as his house, maybe in the same spirit as this selection that is soaked with irony.

Similarly, he seemed to enjoy, in another passage in his journals, describing how once an organization from town held their meeting at his house, more than filling it with their twenty members, like circus clowns in a tiny car.

Expansive and worthwhile ideas need space for discussion. To discuss them effectively, you live in a big way, with adequate imagination and vision. Don't expect inspiring ideas to emerge from a cramped life. But in these matters, irony is often in play. To have a large life you may need a small home.

When, years ago, I was writing about the Marquis de Sade in a favorable way, I was struck by his observation that his prison wardens would have been smart to free him. His cramped prison cell had the effect of liberating his imagination, he said, and therefore he wrote more freely. It's a lesson worth considering: Limitations on your life may make it boundless in areas that really count.

If we are going to speak sincerely and intimately, we need space between us: the space to be individuals and not overly identified with each other. We need to speak softly, not shouting our convictions, if we want to be heard. We may need to stand on opposite sides of a room or lake. We need to enjoy some distance from each other, some separation. Oddly, intimacy sometimes requires room in which to move around.

40

NOT SPIRITUAL, BUT NATURAL

Men nowhere, east or west, live yet a natural life, round which the vine clings, and which the elm willingly shadows. Man would desecrate it by his touch, and so the beauty of the world remains veiled to him. He needs not only to be spiritualized, but naturalized *on the soil of the earth. . . . It is in vain to dream of a wildness distant from ourselves. There is none such. It is the bog in our brain and bowels, the primitive vigor of nature in us, that inspires that dream.*[1]

—Henry David Thoreau, *A Week on the Concord and Merrimack Rivers*

Millions of people today read books, attend workshops, travel to distant parts of the world, and join organizations in a sincere effort to be more spiritual. They look at the world around them and see people doing everything possible to have more possessions and enjoy an overflowing bank account and yearn painfully to be wealthy. These same people, it seems, are dazed by celebrity, a peculiar insanity that seems to suck out one's personal worth. So, it makes sense to turn in the opposite direction and pursue a simpler, less burdened life and aim at a more spiritual, removed, and idealized goal. From the muck of materialism it seems an advance to meditate, pray, and aim for a higher consciousness.

But Thoreau has another idea. In this case, rather than moving upward toward the spiritual, he recommends moving inward to the natural. And not nature as you might expect. You may reconsider the common idea of Thoreau as a naturalist and understand that he is a singular worldly philosopher, or even an artistic psychologist, getting his inspirations outdoors. You will not find the nature you should embrace by looking through a microscope or telescope. These instruments could allow you to peer sharply and deeply into the world, but your perception would be physical and literal. Thoreau wants you discover *your* nature, the secrets of your own reality that you inherit by being human and having your unique existence in the special place destiny has made your home. For Thoreau, nature includes the human being walking the paths and floating the streams. If you want to learn from Thoreau, you might note the point where he moves on from being a naturalist to a natural man.

You live from the bog in your brain and bowels, the primitive vigor of nature in you. Your own mind and gut are the places where you can connect with this aspect of nature. They are the natural life you are hunting for when you paddle your canoe and climb mountains. Thoreau was clear about his life work, as he puts it in famous lines explaining why he spent time at Walden Pond: "I went to the woods because I wished to live deliberately, to front only the essential facts of life." He went to Walden not to be a naturalist, but a person who is truly alive.

I saw my first bog in my early twenties on a dim late evening in County Donegal, Ireland. I have memories of thin shovels slipping with sucking sounds into the wet earth and carving out bricks of peat to be dried and used for fireplaces and ovens. This is Thoreau's image for the natural life in us. We find the bog from which our thoughts emerge and where our damp, underground emotions mix and digest. You may well find the bog when you camp out in nature, but your search is successful only when your campsite lies as much inside you as in the outer world.

I keep saying that Thoreau was not a naturalist, but it would be folly to suggest that he didn't espouse a life in nature. People wonder why he studied nature so closely and yet did not work with his Harvard associates in a more scientific manner. Maybe the difference is that Thoreau consistently understood nature as a doorway to the bog in himself and had in mind to recover and manifest his own reality. Numbers and analyses couldn't grasp what he was after with his toils on rivers and long paths and well-hoed plantings.

You could follow Thoreau literally and paddle a simple boat, canoe, or kayak down a nearby stream, or learn to play a simple flute and see if you can charm the fish or animals. But it might be better to find your own methods that suit you. It would be in the wrong spirit to join a group of Thoreau imitators all playing their flutes on a river.

Thoreau urges us to "see through" the literal realm of nature to its secrets, mysteries, and hidden teachings. If you want to learn from him, notice his intense existential curiosity and emulate his desire to learn what nature had to teach him. We, too, could go beyond tallying data and exploiting nature for products and learn what it teaches us about being human. We could focus, like Thoreau, on the all-important question: To really live and be alive, how should I go about my life?

Most people seem to avoid this question and elect to live in easy unconsciousness. This is exactly what Thoreau did not want. He wanted to live "deliberately," that is, with awareness and choice. He wanted to think through his positions in society and when necessary live in counterpoint to society's values. If it came to that, he would be an eccentric and a gadfly.

To live as an individual in community we, too, may have to discover the bog at the root our feelings and ideas. We may have to examine our emotions and thoughts to be sure they are the ones to live by. It is becoming clear that global suicide is a possibility and maybe inevitable. The reason for this is also becoming clear: mass mental instability. When we are out of touch with our deepest source, we wobble. Then, like most people on the planet, we need psychotherapy.

Leaders around the world have arrived at a point of power where they can act out their sadistic passions for dominance and adulation. These people are clearly grossly immature and profoundly troubled, and yet they gather millions of followers who are drawn into the insanity. If our planet fails, it will be because of emotional illness and severe immaturity. Our real problem is a grand disturbance of soul.

We have a wilderness within, bogs deep in our souls, like Sigmund Freud's id and Carl Jung's unconscious. At the same time these are the source of our raw "material"—our emotions, ideas, impulses, fears, and compulsions. Thoreau's approach to this wild nature in us might give us some hints on how to proceed in a dangerous world. We need not only to become more spiritual in our daily lives but also more natural, more in tune and responsive to the wilderness and the rich muck within us.

Thoreau worked out a way to remain as much as possible in the natural realm outside to benefit from the wildness within. Through sympathetic magic he connected with his inner resources by associating closely with the outer world of nature. We, too, could take seriously our connection to the wild world around us, not just seeing it as a weekend's holiday but as the essential task of our lives, our major route to meaning.

In popular psychology, "personal growth" is taken as an obvious purpose. You never hear of "personal decay." Apparently, we have not learned from nature that growth lasts only a few months before going into decline. We want to be growing constantly, and yet this idea is starkly contrary to nature. Thoreau advises us to know nature well so we can live more naturally, not by having a home in the woods but by having seasons in our lives and periods of both blossom and decay.

When you live your natural life, you do not have to emulate or compete with other people around you. You enjoy both solitude and community in fellowship with people pursuing their own natural lives. You want more community among people going after their own goals, and less conformity. Thoreau cultivated a spiritual life, but he left room for a natural life as well.

41

A RICH AND FERTILE MYSTERY

The scenery, when it is truly seen, reacts on the life of the seer. How to live. How to get the most life. How to extract its honey from the flower of the world. That is my every-day business. I am as busy as a bee about it. I ramble over all fields on that errand, and am never so happy as when I feel myself heavy with honey and wax. I am like a bee searching the livelong day for the sweets of nature . . . .We are surrounded by a rich and fertile mystery. May we not probe it, pry into it, employ ourselves about it, a little? To devote your life to the discovery of the divinity in nature or to the eating of oysters, would they not be attended with very different results?

—Henry David Thoreau, journal entry, September 5, 1851

The water shines with an inward light like a heaven on earth. The silent depth and serenity and majesty of water! Strange that

> *men should distinguish gold and diamonds, when these precious elements are so common.*[1]
>
> ——Henry David Thoreau, journal entry, June 13, 1851

How do you extract honey from the flower of the world? First, you not only look at nature, you really see it. You go out into nature walking, hiking, or boating. You do not study it from a distance. You see with your feet and legs, not just with your eyes. You take it in with all your senses and, as you go, you become more intimate with it, not less so.

Thoreau is in nature like a bee is in a flower—close, active, probing, part of nature, and not observing it from a distance. This closeness has two important consequences: Thoreau sees through the facade of nature to its inherent divinity. His willingness to become intimate with his world allows him to have an immediate experience of the sacred. His walks and paddles bring him close enough to the wildness that he is affected spiritually and theologically. This is the second impact: Thoreau is deeply affected and becomes the person he wants to be.

Our usual way of studying nature gives us a vast supply of information, but it doesn't change us for the better. Our methods leave a gulf between the world and our own lives. We may be affected externally by having more tools and information, but we are not necessarily elevated or transformed. Thoreau says he is as busy as a bee trying to get the most out of life. The wild scenery should "react on the life of the seer."

Scientists could complete their research and inventions by considering how they are affected by their research and then teach us how to live in a society having been instructed by the proximity of the natural world. This must be a planned outcome. Thoreau is a model for artful, conscious living, especially as he valued the place of personal wildness as part of a person's education and maturing.

But how do we get beyond the insufficient information age? In the beginning, Thoreau thought he would be a traditional poet, but he learned that his calling was to be a prose poet, a writer with a subtle, visionary wit. Instead of writing his impressions in verse, he discovered the poetic power of nature, its imagistic and spiritual potency. He changed course and wrote about nature's secrets, its hidden myths, and spiritual powers. He switched from poems to books that combined his observations of nature with his scorching desire to become his own original and natural self. He made every effort to be close to the wilderness, to shape his life accordingly and then to express his developing self in art.

Thoreau kept a journal, a word that means "day." In a journal we go over a day's experience and put those reflections in a special form of language. Less formal and probing, a journal is an opportunity to experiment with language, as Thoreau often does. In his journals you will find alliteration, play on words, etymology, the use of various languages, allusions and references, biblical echoes, mythological motifs, and much more. A journal gave him the freedom to experiment and re-invent himself.

For example, Thoreau doesn't say that the water at Walden Pond is as sacred as the water of the Ganges River in India. He says that the Walden waters *are* the Ganges. Whichever river we float our canoe on is, in fact, the Ganges, or maybe the Euphrates, or Thames, or Liffey. In the passage cited he is more direct than ever: "We are surrounded by a rich and fertile mystery. May we not probe it, pry into it, employ ourselves about it, a little?" I hear a note of sarcasm in that plea. Let's give a *little* attention to the divinity within nature. Maybe it is a little more important than deciding which oysters to eat at dinner.

But we run up against a problem that Emerson and Thoreau both faced: Their idea of religion went against the prevailing practice of the society in which they lived. Given his radical ideas, Emerson felt he had to leave the ministry he had prepared for shortly after beginning it, because his own thought had drifted away from tradition. Like Thoreau looking for signs of divinity in nature, Emerson wanted a direct experience of the divine. In his Divinity School address at Harvard in 1838, he said to the scholars and students around him, "Let me admonish you, first of all, to go alone; to refuse the good models, even those which are sacred in the imagination of men, and dare to love God without mediator or veil."[2]

"We are surrounded by a rich and fertile mystery," Thoreau adds. The trees and rocks and waters have a presence. If you have the eyes and ears for it, you will sense an invisible potency in nature that affects you and often resets your life and gives you focus. Wonder deeply and seriously about it. Give it your attention. Ultimately, dedicate your life to it.

This dedication can become a new form of religion, in the best and deepest sense of the word. Not just a belief system or a collection of moral rules, but your way of relating to life's inherent mysteries. Nature is then not a reservoir of raw materials for making the materialistic world, but a container of mysteries and meanings. In a letter written when Thoreau was two years old, John Keats wrote to his brother: "Call the world if you Please 'The vale of Soul-making.'"[3]

Nature points beyond itself, as when we stand on a dark night looking at the stars. Naturally we wonder what it is all about and how we are connected to that vast mysterious space. You can have the same transportive experience watching a bee do its work in a flower or just wondering about the rain and how it affects how you feel and how you interpret your experience. You can learn from the rain to be fresh, renewed, cleansed, and made fertile.

Thoreau suggests that we take some time to reach beyond ourselves and capture the eternal realities that lie deep within the world and yet are infinitely close to our own lives. Here, the poetic and the spiritual join forces and together invent a new kind of religion, transcendence within the ordinary and everyday. Emerson suggested noticing the miracle of rain as a step toward a more immediate religious experience. Thoreau did not use such language, but admitted to being a natural yogi. His practice was to walk without a plan, make friends with animals, and find his entertainment in nature.

The idea is to look closely and with a friendly eye at the familiar things of nature and see beyond them to the meanings they contain. If you look deep enough, with enough reverence for nature's secrets, you will catch a glimpse of the nameless and the infinite. It is not only up in the sky, but close at hand on the bush and in the stream. Thoreau constantly writes about this kind of seeing, and he never pauses from doing it.

42

SOUL SCULPTING

Every man is the builder of a temple, called his body, to the god he worships, after a style purely his own, nor can he get off by hammering marble instead. We are all sculptors and painters, and our material is our own flesh and blood and bones. Any nobleness begins at once to refine a man's features, any meanness or sensuality to imbrute them.[1]

—Henry David Thoreau, *Walden*

These words of Henry David Thoreau are reminiscent of a well-known passage from Plotinus, the third century C.E. founder of Neoplatonism and forerunner of soul studies: "Withdraw into yourself and look. And if you do not find yourself beautiful yet, act as does the creator of a statue that is to be made beautiful: he cuts away here, he smoothes there, he makes this line lighter, this other purer, until a lovely face has grown upon his work. So do you also: cut away all that is excessive, straighten all that is crooked, bring light to all that is overcast, labour to make all one glow of beauty and never cease chiselling your statue."[2]

The aim of life is to craft the soul from nature and from the raw materials we find in and around us. How we use those materials determines the shape of our souls and whether they are beautiful. Both Plotinus and Keats felt that the primary aim in life is not meaning but beauty. Today people seem more interested in a healthy life than a beautiful one, but maybe we should follow Thoreau and aim for nobility of character.

Today, people want information and entertainment. Plotinus, Keats, and Thoreau are seeking something else as their goal. They want to experience the fullness of life, and Thoreau in particular, following his friend Emerson, wants to be an individual, and to that end he practiced self-culture. He was determined to craft his person and his life. We come back to his phrase "to live deliberately," which has perhaps more force than the modern idea of living "consciously."

Keats famously wrote to a friend saying, "What the imagination seizes as Beauty must be truth."[3] We might say that our goal is to live with grace and awareness. The primary goal is aesthetics, not health. A person who is physically ill or emotionally off-center might still be beautiful. Thoreau learned from his reading in Eastern spirituality that to be beautiful is to follow your dharma, the rule of your own life—to live with intention and design. You uncover the truth of your reality, and the resulting life is beautiful. Maybe this is why, in his last sermon, the Buddha held up a flower for all to contemplate. His final word had to do with natural beauty.

Life is always difficult, but its beauty could be found in satisfying work, having good people as friends, and in activities that engage talents for service and creativity. When Thoreau moved out to Walden, spent a night in jail, climbed Monadnock and took risks for the Underground Railroad, he was sculpting his life and making it art. We make an art of life by making good decisions and acting on them.

These moments make us, for better or worse, unique. When these actions give birth to virtues such as justice, generosity, empathy, kindness, service, and guidance, there emerges a perfected existence, a life that may be difficult in some ways and yet beautiful.

The word *perfect* does not have to mean without fault, but rather "lived through to the end." You sense beauty in a person when you perceive a life fully lived. A beautified human being has not refused opportunities for fulfillment. Instead of avoiding life, they have fulfilled it and brought it to a point of excellence, an outcome the ancient Greeks called arete, the completion of what is possible.

From these two writers, Keats and Thoreau, we have the central and rich idea that soul is to be crafted with aesthetic values. Thoreau warns against letting your way of life "imbrute" you, dehumanize you. This is a word we could use more often, becoming aware of those things that denude us of our civilization and take away our refinement.

Thoreau crafts his soul, and that opus is the heart of my dialogue with him in this book. He had a unique way of soulmaking, a method that we can make our own, with our individual differences. We certainly do not have to imitate him in his outward lifestyle, but we can adopt his principles and even some of his quirks. We could reflect on his unique ways of interpreting the natural world around him, discovering ways to be original and even eccentric. Instead of risking imbrutement, we could find pleasure in the opposite direction of perfected, beautiful character.

When you look at our world today, you can see many striking examples of natural beauty, where nature is still intact and accessible. But ugliness abounds where architecture is cheap and unimaginative, and functional without real concern for beauty. Human life still struggles in search of peace, care, and dignity. Most people do not have an Emerson nearby to teach and guide them, giving them a vital and optimistic philosophy of life. Most still live under a religious canopy of fear and demand, and few can alternate, as Thoreau did, between pure nature and human culture. Most have not yet discovered the joy of a beautiful life.

Above all, we need to be psychologically mature and have clear and open hearts. Today we are so accustomed to guile in leadership that we cannot imagine life without it. Guile is sleight-of-hand deceit, a habit of concealing one's intentions. His neighbors complained of Thoreau's many shortcomings, but they never accused him of guile.

Thoreau uses the word *nobleness*, where we might say *nobility*. It is the virtue that ultimately gives us the beauty of character we are after. Friedrich Nietzsche describes nobility as "a divining of values for which scales have not yet been invented: a sacrificing on altars which are consecrated to an unknown God: a bravery without the desire for honor."[4] It is an elevation of the person to a special level of sensitivity and magnanimity. The word *noble* comes from an Indo-European root that means "to know how to live." It is the opposite of guile, which is planted in ignorance. Thoreau wanted to live a noble life, exalted without the imbruting element of narcissistic self-advancement.

To develop nobility of character you need good teaching and a community of elevated people to show you how to do it. Parents could model it for their children and teachers could put it in their curriculum. Each of us could learn from Thoreau how to find our path to excellence of character from the world around us. *Deliberate* may be the key word. We may have to be more deliberate about soulmaking and character building.

I have had models of nobility in my life, and they have guided me. One was Father Gregory O'Brien, a priest who was my high school English teacher. He brought remarkable character and vitality into an otherwise sleepy school. He was a torch, full of heat and light, who taught my mates and me the importance of wit and solid humor and study and art. I was transformed by his presence and by his special attention to me and my progress toward an elusive maturity.

When I worked for a short time at a Catholic church leading adult education programs, I had a colleague, a nun, Sister Betty Foster, who was a no-nonsense, deeply caring, selfless, and intelligent woman. We would often attend boring and useless meetings, and Betty would be sitting apart from me. At key moments she would take out a beautiful, leather-wrapped letter opener in the form of a Spanish dagger and, just for my benefit, "stab" herself with it, expressing her frustration with the inanity around us. One day she gave me that dagger, and I still have it on my desk as I write, reminding me of her as a woman of immense nobility and fun, her memory telling me never to be boring.

Nobility does not have to be stuffy and excessively high-minded. But it is an elevation of character that requires a degree of moral loftiness. You rise to its demands and its pleasures. We learn from the learned, gifted, and humble Thoreau how to aim high and become comfortable with a sculpted character that is not ruined by self-interest.

43

SLIGHT IMPULSES

You will spend this afternoon in setting up your neighbor's stove, and be paid for it. I will spend it gathering the few berries of the vaccinium Oxycoccus which Nature produces here, before it is too late, and be paid for it also after another fashion. I have always reaped unexpected and incalculable advantages from carrying out at last, however tardily, any little enterprise which my genius suggested to me long ago as a thing to be done,—some step to be taken, however slight, out of the usual course.

It is these comparatively cheap and private expeditions that substantiate our existence and batten our lives, as, where a vine touches the earth in its undulating course, it puts forth roots and thickens its stock. Our employment generally is tinkering, mending the old worn-out teapot of society. Our stock in trade is solder. Better for me, says my genius, to go cranberrying this afternoon for the Vaccinium Oxycoccus in Gowing's Swamp, to get but a pocketful and learn its peculiar flavor, aye, and the flavor of Gowing's Swamp and of life in New

> *England, than go consul to Liverpool and get I don't know how many thousands of dollars for it, with no such flavor.*[1]
>
> —Henry David Thoreau, journal entry, August 30, 1856

Better to taste a common cranberry in our hand, says Henry David Thoreau, than to become an official in Liverpool, England, as Nathaniel Hawthorne, Thoreau's friend and neighbor, did. It's especially important to pay attention to the smallest impulses toward some action or experiment in life that comes to us or may be a long-held practice. These simple impulses take us deeper into life than grand appointments and positions.

This does not mean that a great adventure will not give us a boost and a taste of what we can become, but the tiny urges are also valuable for seeding the self. Thoreau compares these small indications to a vine that touches the ground and takes root. It's a subtle comparison and a striking image for how we "grow." Thoreau's image for a successful life is not a tall commanding tree but an almost invisible vine hidden among branches touching the earth and taking root.

Some small inspirations fade in time, while others scrape the ground and are fertile. For me, one such commonplace ingredient to the growing of a self was the tradition my family had of traveling in the summers from Detroit, where we lived, to rural New York State, where my grandmother's brothers had a 125-acre farm. Once there, you would think you were living in the nineteenth century, with the weathered barn and seemingly ancient outbuildings and the emotionally warm but physically lacking farmhouse that had no running water, limited electricity, and the musty smell of decades of bachelor brothers living mainly in the old kitchen with its well-trodden linoleum floor.

I could have been at home in a more modern setting, but the simple life on a farm suited me at the time, and I didn't mind the spider- and bumble bee–infested outhouse. Some summers I spent entirely on this farm with my old diabetic Aunt Kitty, who daily asked me to take care of her chamber pot. This simple living gave me the building blocks of my character.

The old-fashioned farm life was not much different from the life Thoreau cites as offering "incalculable advantages." I carry that farm with me even now in my old age. It keeps me grounded and somewhat simple and always at home in nature. Sometimes I wish that I had been born into a more ambitious and highly educated family, but then I remember how my warm and homely background gave me the plainer and deeper qualities that have guided my life work.

You could follow Thoreau's unusual advice by placing more weight on ordinary experiences that shape you than on extravagant wishes for a highly placed origin. When you think about who you want to be, consider the deeper inclinations that are plain rather than exciting. Even if one day you reach for the stars, these humble elements may, in the long run, give you more than the more sophisticated experiences of education and travel. They reach further into character and give you a depth that affects your relationships and achievements.

I have had two close friends who worked in inner-city hospitals and cared seriously about the impoverished people who lived in the neighborhood. One was Dr. Joel Elkes, a pioneer in drug therapies for mentally ill patients, and the other the Reverend Marcus McKinney, who is dedicated to bringing soul to medicine. They both put their careers on the line to help the people they saw out of the corner of their eyes. Their fellow doctors wanted them to develop national and even international programs for the advancement of hospitals. But my friends couldn't get past the images they had in their minds of poor people living near their hospitals who needed care.

This more personal, less adventurous, and programmatic focus I think is what Thoreau was talking about. These humbler goals will offer you an individual experience of life and a rich and deeply etched identity. Don't give in to the flashier alternatives that are not you, that have not snuck into you. Learn the difference between worldly success and self-unfolding. Do not lose sight of the value of small goals and low horizons.

Thoreau's way to stay close to the path given him by his nature and fate was to remember projects that came to him long ago, resurrect them, and fulfill those impulses to move further into himself. Invariably, those projects would be simple in comparison to his neighbors' efforts, like picking berries rather than fixing a stove for profit. Typically, Thoreau's forays into nature are not for the sensation of cash in the pocket, but rather the taste of a fresh-picked berry. Also, his projects tended to be outside the normal. It is worth including that value in our own ways of spending time. Do not do what is expected or usual. The very oddness of the job might give it some importance in the manifestation of your individual personality.

Some, I know, distrust Ralph Waldo Emerson, Henry David Thoreau, and Walt Whitman, even Emily Dickinson, for not being social enough. *Self-reliance*, that term that Emerson clung to, may sound selfish and self-centered. But it may be only the beginning, the first phase, followed by community. Emerson was constantly in touch with people, helping them get along, as when he permitted Thoreau to use his land at Walden Pond and when he guided Nathaniel Hawthorne, Bronson Alcott, Margaret Fuller, and many others, when he stood strong for abolition and traveled often to spread the word about a new American intelligence. He made efforts to entice people to move to Concord to create an American community.

My childhood taste of farm living formed me and gave me an appreciation for the simple life, the natural world, animals, the seasons, the weather, and hard work. I came to love the animals, the skillful attention of horses, the lightness of oats, and the multitude of creatures in the pasture's winding creek. Following Thoreau's idea, I can take that early experience as a seed for who I am and build on it, noticing where my life today, which is quite different, might benefit from those memories and learnings. I could return to sensations of the simple life, not so dependent on machines and conveniences.

In Thoreau's spirit, I could give my own life a special quality by drawing on my early farm experiences without any desire to convert others to these values. I could do it quietly and somewhat privately and see if my life might be enriched by this farm tendril catching in the earth of my being. I could choose a few more exciting and exotic experiences as main sources of character, but navigating an outhouse is a skill worth preserving.

In the quoted passage, Thoreau says that this could be a step taken "however slight, out of the usual course." Try to picture the dynamics here. You take a slight step out of your usual pattern, dipping into some past experience or learning, and move more deeply into yourself, living now more as you, rather than as someone highly influenced by family or culture. You may link to something in your past, like my farm days, or to a minor impulse to do something out of character or your normal practice.

Thoreau's suggestion removes the heroic from our wish to make a meaningful, individual life. The heroic pattern of setting goals, overcoming obstacles, and staying on course is the mythology of our time, so unconscious as to be unnoticed as it consumes our energies. Everything we "tackle" in our ordinary lives becomes a "battle" to "overcome," an "enemy," whether it is cancer, drugs, poverty, or prejudice.

Thoreau, ever the nonhero, not even bold enough to be named an antihero, gives us this useful insight: The small, special moments in your life, not obviously central or significant, may be the seeds of a potent and creative future.

44

ON TIPTOE

The works of the great poets have never yet been read by mankind, for only great poets can read them. They have only been read as the multitude read the stars, at most astrologically, not astronomically. Most men have learned to read to serve a paltry convenience, as they have learned in cipher in order to keep accounts and not be cheated in trade; but of reading as a noble intellectual exercise they know little or nothing; yet this only is reading in a high sense, not that which lulls us as a luxury and suffers the nobler faculties to sleep the while, but what we have to stand on tip-toe to read and devote our most alert and wakeful hours to.

I think that having learned our letters we should read the best that is in literature, and not be forever repeating our a b abs, and words of one syllable, in the fourth or fifth classes, sitting on the lowest and foremost form, all our lives.[1]

—Henry David Thoreau, *Walden*

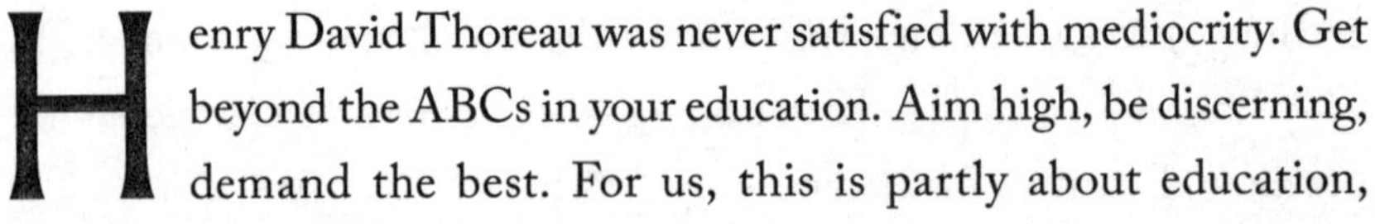

Henry David Thoreau was never satisfied with mediocrity. Get beyond the ABCs in your education. Aim high, be discerning, demand the best. For us, this is partly about education, learning the most culture has to offer, but it is also about the quality of our daily lives: how we spend our time, who we read and listen to, what movies we watch, how we get our news and analysis. Today we are not only what we read but who and what we expose ourselves to.

The average person doesn't want a fussy, self-important society, but we can have quality of thought and cultural experience without class-dominated superiority. Thoreau shunned polite society, yet he consistently advocated for the noblest kind of learning. He was rough around the edges, but he was also well-read and deeply reflective. Around ideas, he did not take the easy, well-trod path. He was a self-professed clodhopper and a full-muddied scholar.

The world today is in serious trouble. Our problems are deep and complex. They require stellar language, profound ideas, a schooled imagination, a sophisticated playful spirit, and an honest, unaligned, natural way to be spiritual. We are usually satisfied, in the matters that mean the most, with the average and the good enough. We seem threatened with quality of thought, the far reach of ideas and ideals, the demands of a sterling moral life, and the far depth of genuine religious or spiritual insight.

Our biggest problem is the continuing secularization of a sacred planet. The paradox is that the more religion becomes rigid and fanatical, the more secular the world becomes. One supports the other. For they are extremes: secularism and religious fanaticism. When do you ever hear an open-minded, truly probing theological conversation? Rarely. Yet nothing could be more important than to hone our ideas about morality, contemplation, and meaning in the universe and in our own lives. *Science* used to mean "knowledge" or "knowing." Now it refers to technical, empirical analysis. Today, even science could be taken deeper, beyond technical and informational sophistication to wonder about our lives and our future, a spiritual pursuit as well as a physical one.

Does the average person need access to great ideas presented in golden language? Or are standard, unremarkable language and ideas sufficient? At Gettysburg, should Abraham Lincoln have said, "Eighty-seven years ago our leaders set up a new country on the ideals of liberty and equality"? Or, "Four score and seven years ago our fathers brought forth on this continent, a new nation, conceived in liberty, and dedicated to the proposition that all men are created equal." William Shakespeare's Hamlet says, "To be or not to be, that is the question." Should he have said, "Should I live or die, that's what I'm wondering"? The loss of manners and formalities makes for a crude society that tries to progress on below-standard habits and mere casual language.

It is entirely short-sighted to use loose language for a formal event, and it is equally misguided to be formal at an ordinary occasion. It is all about culture, which is cultus, a way to allow ordinary and simple rituals to carry the weight of our lives. Speaking with each other is a form of ritual that could benefit from occasional and easy formality.

Consistent with Thoreau's habit of seeing through the literal facade of things to their more meaningful and sacred nature, we could look more deeply into the connection between *cult* and *culture*. The *American Heritage Dictionary* defines *cult* as "an extreme religious sect living in an unconventional manner under a charismatic leader." That is one kind of cult, and one that most people probably think of when they hear the word. But those of us who study world religions carefully know that *cult* also means "a formal way of expressing religious reverence."

Similarly, culture is life refined through craft, ideas, and imagination. Formality and manners, cult as ritual, assist us when as strangers we try to work together and agree on projects. Culture is not raw, but cooked with rites, special language, and art. If you look closely at the creations of culture, you may find vestiges of religious actions and images. Thoreau does this when he speaks of bathing as a sacrament and rising early as his yoga practice and his explorations in nature as looking for divinity. He looks at the secular and sees the sacred. His quest for the divine undergirds his attempt to create a meaningful life.

Today we think that reading is mainly for information. In books we search for facts and are impressed with the results of numerical studies of behavior. We trust numbers and are impressed with authors who can cite study after study, seemingly proving their ideas by making sums and analyzing data. But this is not the kind of reading Thoreau advocates. He describes good reading as "noble intellectual enterprise." We need to read books that demand that we stand on tiptoe to reach them. We read beyond ourselves, not beneath ourselves.

Today there are many ways beyond books to ennoble our minds and hearts. With e-readers, technology has made reading more accessible and convenient. Even writing gets a boost from text messages and emails that at least invite us to express ourselves in words. The book is still an excellent technology. You can carry it and pack it easily and discover ideas and art in all its pages. It can be nonfiction, fiction, or poetry, and it can inspire and refine. It can humanize.

Thoreau's advice is crucial: Don't settle for the least and lowest in life. Read what is worth your while. Know the difference between a glut of words and literature. Know how to distinguish a writer from an author. I say, read equal amounts of fiction, prose, and poetry. How else to say it, don't waste your precious time on anything beneath you. Don't be too fussy, but don't sink too low.

Thoreau was not the great intellectual or a typical philosopher. He was grounded in his thought by hoeing beans and wading in swamps. And yet he always recommends reaching high and doing everything, including reading, at a level of quality. We could follow him in this, having the richest ideas even as we live our ordinary lives. It's an interesting ideal: Read only the best books, only those worthy of you and able to elevate your life. At the same time find joy in gardening, hiking, and traipsing in mud. Become a passionate intellectual, but do not give up your animal spirit.

45

A VILLAGE A UNIVERSITY

We have a comparatively decent system of common schools for infants only; but excepting the half-starved Lyceum in the winter, and latterly the puny beginning of a library suggested by the State, no school for ourselves. We spend more on almost any article of bodily aliment or ailment than on our mental aliment. It is time we had uncommon schools, that we did not leave off our education when we begin to be men and women. It is time that villages were universities, and their elder inhabitants the fellows of universities, with leisure—if they are indeed so well off—to pursue liberal studies the rest of their lives. Shall the world be confined to one Paris or one Oxford forever? Cannot students be boarded here and get a liberal education under the skies of Concord? Can we not hire some Abelard to lecture to us? . . . That is the uncommon school we want . . . If it is necessary, omit one bridge over the river, go round a little there, and throw one arch at least over the darker gulf of ignorance which surrounds us.[1]

—Henry David Thoreau, *Walden*

This passionate paragraph from *Walden* is not just about what we call adult education, but about the idea of learning and studying all our lives and not seeing school as being relevant only to children. The word *school* comes the Latin word *schola*, which means "leisure," and Henry David Thoreau says that the leisure we have when life is good allows us to learn more as adults. Today, it seems, leisure is treated as a time for passive entertainment, which is certainly a worthy aim, but we need not divide life into work and entertainment. Leisure is also for learning.

Learning is different from education, which we usually see as a public process in which one highly informed person presents their knowledge to others. Today we imagine being educated as a means for making money. We reward those who have passed through our educational system with degrees, certificates, and credentials. The education they have "received" allows them to advance socially and financially.

But learning is not a system. A person may successfully complete their education without learning much, and certainly without becoming a learned person. Learning is the individual person's advance in knowledge, seen from the person rather than the system. Learning has little to do with making money or job training. It is not even about acquiring information and skills, but about becoming a mature, sophisticated, and thoughtful person. If you say a person is learned, you don't mean that they have good skills and know plenty of facts. You mean that this person has become remarkable for their interior life, for having the capacity to think and to enrich their thought with references to other learned people.

As usual, Thoreau doesn't just present the prosaic idea that we need education all our lives; he says a village should hire a Peter Abelard, a celebrated medieval teacher and thinker at the University of Paris, to guide the learning of ordinary citizens. Thoreau is taking the idea of lifelong learning to a high pitch. Don't build that bridge you think your town needs; rather, use the money to hire an Abelard, an ideal superior teacher. Make the learning in your town uncommon, not the lowest common denominator. Aim high. Try to create a learned and intellectually sophisticated citizenry. Make your town a patron of the fine arts. Make it a hotbed of rich ideas.

I know, it's easy for me to propose Thoreau's ideal. He was a Harvard graduate, and I have had the opportunity to have an education in the classics and the arts. These two eggheads, Thoreau and Moore, would like a society made up of people who love to read and study. We are suggesting that you and your "village" understand the importance of learning as a proper and necessary way to be human. You cannot solve society's problems with a shallow education; we all need to be learned people.

I propose some nourishing ideas—or, as Thoreau would say, an aliment—some food for our souls, an antidote to the soulless society we have been creating with our runaway machinery and quantified ways of analyzing our experience. A good aliment for our minds and hearts would be a village or society that would provide the tools and teachers for every citizen to keep learning the whole of their life, especially learning about life and how to live a rich and meaningful one.

If you stop learning, you are not only mind dead but also soul dead. The mind is an activity of the soul that keeps it on the right track and gives it the nourishment that would offer both meaning and pleasure, two of the most important experiences in a life. If there is one thing that is inhibiting humanity from creating a sustaining culture, it is weakening intelligence. We need to be intelligent practically, spiritually, aesthetically, and scientifically, but it would take a revolution in culture, some future education age, parallel to the information age, to make our villages universities.

Imagine if your city or town would take on the task of providing learning for its people, inviting the best speakers to visit and speak to the people in an attractive and compelling setting. The lyceum of Thoreau's day, for all the lack of financial support Thoreau complains about, at least was a forum for serious learning and conversation among citizens. Thoreau's mentor and friend Ralph Waldo Emerson gave many of those talks, and he took seriously his role as teacher of the commons and cultivated his role of public speaker and public teacher. Others in their circle did the same, giving themselves to their teaching. Margaret Fuller, friend and colleague to both Emerson and Thoreau, in Boston, offered conversations for women on mythology and other enriching topics.

Emerson had a special form of dress for his lectures, and he says he spent twenty-one hours preparing each one. For the transcendentalists of his time, he was Abelard, a visiting speaker from the blue ethereal realms, and people gathered in numbers to hear him. They came for both enjoyment and learning, as Emerson, and later Thoreau, stood before the crowds in the embodiment of their purpose: to inspire learning and serious discussion among fellow citizens.

We don't have many lyceums today, and in our electronic world we probably wouldn't expect live lectures, maybe not lectures at all, since we are less formal in almost all forms of gathering. But it may be worth our while to reconsider restricting learning to the university or college. If we were to reintroduce lectures in our towns, they would have to be more engaging and not partisan. We can do them online, but Thoreau's idea is to have each village offer a live occasion of learning.

As an author who has published over thirty books, I have been on many book tours. I've stood in front of crowds, some small and some shockingly large, engaging people in the pursuit of rich ideas. I know that we can turn our cities and towns into universities—that is a metaphor—places of learning and advancement in character.

Once, I was lecturing at a church in Dallas, Texas, a "village" I knew well. After describing an approach to the spiritual that would be deep and open-minded, I offered a challenge to the city. Dallas is known as a business town deep into the pursuit of wealth, the epitome of materialism. To the few hundred citizens sitting in front of me, I said with some passion: "Work at it. Make Dallas the center of a world-wide spiritual renewal, a Mecca for anyone seeking profound wisdom. Think of Tibet and the Dalai Lama. Not sectarian self-protective belief, but the center of a wide-ranging, intense spiritual learning and practice."

I wanted to challenge a city I loved, as its citizens sat in front of me. That is one way to follow through on Thoreau's idea of making a village a university. Another way is for a city or town to establish a relationship with a lecturer or a group to visit the city regularly to support its learning activities. Thoreau suggests getting the best teachers possible from anywhere in the world and trade a big development project for a special opportunity for learning. Think of your own town or city as one big university. What would it look like? What would it be like to be a citizen there?

46

THE WALDEN POND SOCIETY

About a month ago, at the post-office, Abel Brooks, who is pretty deaf, sidling up to me, observed in a loud voice which all could hear, "Let me see, your society is pretty large, Ain't it?" "Oh, yes, large enough," said I, not knowing what he meant. "There's Stewart belongs to it, and Collier, he's one of them and Emerson, and my boarder" (Pulsifer), "and Channing, I believe, I think he goes there." "You mean the walkers; *don't you?" "Ye-es, I call you the Society. All go to the woods; don't you?" "Do you miss any of your wood?" I asked. "No, I hain't worried any yet. I believe you're a pretty clever set, as good as the average," et., etc.*

Telling Sanborn of this, he said that, when he came to town and boarded at Holbrook's, he asked H. how many religious societies there were in town. H. said that there were three,—the Unitarian, the Orthodox, and the Walden Pond Society.[1]

—Henry David Thoreau, journal entry, April 16, 1857

One important theme in Henry David Thoreau's retreat to Walden Pond is the making of a new kind of religion and a new approach to the spiritual life. According to his story, in Concord, Massachusetts, there were three religions: the Unitarian, the established churches, and the Walden Pond Society. Ralph Waldo Emerson, William Ellery Channing, Thoreau, and their friends constituted a new kind of religion that they called transcendentalism, for which did not have a definite doctrine but focused on a few values:

1. To explore a transcendent realm beyond human limits but do so without formal religion or the traditional language.
2. To find new ways to educate, like not using intimidation or being limited to intellectual learning.
3. To establish a relationship with the natural world and discover it as a major source of self-understanding.
4. To complete any learning and insights by expressing them in poetry or some other art.
5. To study, read, and have serious public and private conversations around a meaningful and creative existence.
6. To keep in mind the value of the individual person, not in contrast to community, but important in itself.
7. To create a uniquely American philosophy and lifestyle.

The transcendentalists would often meet in Boston, but frequently they came to live in, or at least visit, Concord. In Thoreau's time there was a train running between the big city and the smaller town. But sometimes these high-minded thinkers would take a horse and buggy or just walk the eighteen-mile distance, about a six-hour walk. They would meet in each other's houses and often stop at Emerson's house or give a talk at a lyceum meeting. Bronson Alcott liked to have "conversations," somewhat formal discussions of points he prepared ahead of time. Thoreau preferred to go on long walks with people, climb mountains, or go out on a boat. One of his regular companions was William Ellery Channing, a talented transcendentalist who was married to Margaret Fuller's sister.

Emerson owned fourteen acres at Walden Pond and would walk contemplatively in those woods, as Thoreau's quaint story describes. He and his friends were the informal Walden Pond Society, an alternative to the Unitarians or the usual churchgoers.

This group is particularly relevant to us today because they were cultivating a spiritual way of life without the trappings of organized religion. Many today are looking for something similar. Nature was their source, as laid out in Emerson's important essay of that name. There he writes: "In the woods, we return to reason and faith. There I feel that nothing can befall me in life,—no disgrace, no calamity, (leaving me my eyes,) which nature cannot repair. Standing on the bare ground,—my head bathed by the blithe air, and uplifted into infinite space,—all mean egotism vanishes. I become a transparent eye-ball; I am nothing; I see all; the currents of the Universal Being circulate through me; I am part or particle of God."

This essay was a starting point for Thoreau, as it could be for you and me. It brings centuries of mysticism into our own time, made available to us, and it all begins in nature, in a simple walk in the woods. Another frequent theme of Thoreau: simplicity. He makes a point that their walk did no harm to the woods, and the neighbor understands that it was a religious experience, even if he did not get the full significance of transcendentalism.

Egotism goes away in the woods, and the walkers may have a transcendent experience, finding themselves "uplifted into infinite space."

Emerson had read Neoplatonists, who believed that we are saturated with divine being, and Eastern philosophies, which taught similar mystical views. But they all, especially Thoreau, practiced it in simple ways, starting with direct experiences in the natural world. Thoreau's journal entries are about eighty percent observations of nature and the rest reflections on how to live from your innermost being. Simplicity all around.

At this time in my life I live in the New Hampshire woods on a small pond—my own Walden. One of my favorite moments of meditation happens when I sit back on a chair at my house and look up at the tops of tall oak trees between me and the lake. I see how they change with the seasons and how they sashay in the wind and how birds of all sizes arrive and perch on their very tops. In strong winds the trees blow and howl. Last summer a small tornado blew in from Mount Monadnock and across the pond and up onto our beachfront, taking out several trees and battering my aluminum rowboat.

As a monk in my youth I spent thirteen years meditating while sitting in silence, hoping to clear my mind of everything. Today I prefer to *contemplate*, a word closer to my practice than *meditate*, under the canopy of trees and within reach of the pond. I prefer the variety of nature's conditions and the sensuous awareness of its presence and its impact on me. When I contemplate the world, I am including it in my sense of self, and asking to be invited into its secret society. I am more me when the natural world is present to my identity. I am bigger in scope—though less, as Emerson promises—egotistical.

We could all exchange vacant worship attendance, if that is our experience, for our own Walden Pond Society, using our own appropriate name from the nature around us. I might call mine Squantum Pond Society, after the Native American man Tisqantum (Squanto), who helped the European settlers when they arrived on Plymouth Bay.

We could have friends of a common vision with whom we can walk in enchanted woods, the simplicity and ordinariness of which are part of its potency. We might rediscover the deep joy of our own spiritual path, our own tending of the great mysteries that leads to a vast expansion and focus of self and community. Following Thoreau's lead, we could discover our own natural religion and a natural self.

47

WHAT MAKES ME RICH

It is foolish for a man to accumulate material wealth chiefly, houses and land. Our stock in life, our real estate, is that amount of thought which we have had, which we have thought out. The ground we have thus created is forever pasturage for our thoughts. I fall back on to visions which I have had. What else adds to my possessions and makes me rich in all lands? If you have ever done any work with these finest tools, the imagination and fancy and reason, it is a new creation, independent on the world, and a possession forever. You have laid up something against a rainy day. You have to that extent cleared the wilderness.

—Henry David Thoreau, journal entry, May 1, 1857

It is a certain faeryland where we live. You may walk out in any direction over the earth's surface lifting your horizon, and everywhere your path, climbing the convexity of the globe, leads you between heaven and earth, not away from the light of the sun and stars and the habitations of men. I wonder that I ever get five miles on my way, the walk is so crowded with events and phenomena. How many questions there are which I have not put to the inhabitants.[1]

—Henry David Thoreau, journal entry, June 7, 1851

What is the nature of wealth? What makes us truly rich? What is it that is worth slaving for and piling up and cashing in after a life of toil? Is it a house, a car, stocks, an IRA? Henry David Thoreau offers another answer to that standing question: It is the ideas we have had and the things we have thought through. It is whatever we have created with imagination, fantasy, and mind. It is something apart from the actual world. It is our own collection of interior things that we keep on shelves in the mind and in a private attic of the heart.

Over time we create a rich treasure of the mind, and we have cleared land in our soul where our singular lives can grow. Piling up these creations is a lifelong work, and at each stage we can take advantage of what we have accumulated. What we have read, too, remains in us like money in the bank. We can rely on and build on it, developing an intelligence that allows us to live deeply and successfully. In a world short on good ideas, it may sound odd to say that our wealth depends on them.

I have never lost the love of study I learned in my early years as a monk. Monks have always been scholars, and they are usually pictured with books, libraries, and calligraphy. Today I may not read all the many books I have stacked in my house, but the presence of a library encourages me not only to read, and thus build up the territory of my imagination, but to create an atmosphere of study.

Walk into a house without a library, and you sense the absence of one of the essentials of life. I know that I am writing as an old person about a former time, but I am sure we can find a way to keep a library in the digital era. The best way might be to do both: use e-readers and maintain a private physical library. Buy an electronic tablet, but do not get rid of your books.

Without books, or their equivalent, we are left in the wilderness of a society dedicated only to entertainment and labor. We work hard and then seek out delicious stupor in entertainment. Enter a house that has books on its walls, and you have entered a sanctum. It is holy like a church, a sanctuary of the imagination. Books are not just sources of information, they are a symbolic presence signifying learning and wisdom.

Once you place books on a shelf, you have made a library, which is not an orderly collection of books but a vision that speaks to the soul. It is like a side altar in a church or temple. That library makes your home different and set apart from your culture, which is dedicated to the world outside rather than the one that Teresa of Ávila described as an "interior castle." It only takes three books to make a basic library, but they need a shelf. Arrange them so they create a book atmosphere. Thoreau liked both an external library and an internal one.

The inner world of meaning complements the external world of objects and actions. In the inner pasture we graze on our own ideas and reflections that have gathered over a lifetime. We reflect on our experiences in accordance with our interpretations and ideas. Through this process of digesting our thoughts and experiences, we become persons.

The person who does not study has nothing of real value to talk about, because life is not only action and experience but also ideas and narratives. You live, and then you store up and process what you have lived. That process is fertilized by ideas and other cultured means of reflection. If you have no ideas, all you can do is repeat the literal stories. You are not only boring, you are vacant.

Ideas do not have to be highly abstract, dry, and distant. They can be rich, and you can come to love them and associate them with you. You may take them from others, especially the giants of literature, but you can make them your own by gathering them in your own way and expressing them in language suited to you. Think of them as bespoke concepts that reside in your home.

Instead of living the usual pattern of action and rest, you might go from experience to reflection. You process your experiences and eventually transmute them into ideas that you can clarify, compare, define, and exchange. Thinking deeply and exchanging your thoughts with others is a major part of being human. It gives your life value. Without it, you are only half a person.

You can engage in this essential processing of events in many other ways: writing poems, keeping a journal, writing letters, taking photos, creating songs and visual images, painting, dancing. Thoreau uses the image of a pasture: treating the environment as food. You graze on the world and absorb it all as you sustain yourself.

In your initial processing of events you are laying something up for a rainy day, giving a raw event a form that you can retain and come back to for further ruminating. Conversation is a powerful means of reflection, and is one that Bronson Alcott, a friend of both Emerson and Thoreau, used as his main method of teaching. Real conversation, not the gossiping that Thoreau complained about as the main preoccupation of his town. I often suggest to people wanting more depth to take any conversation they are in one step deeper. Take the risk. If you sense the shallowness of your interchange, be strong. Take the leap and make your conversation richer.

Alcott was notoriously poor for most of his life, and yet he was rich in ideas and visions for a human future. He traveled often to lead conversations on ideas about an elevated life. He also explored fresh and humane ways to teach children. In his sheer humanity, he was a wealthy man. Alcott said of Thoreau that he was "a sylvan man accomplished in the virtues of an aboriginal civility, and quite superior to the urbanities of cities."[2] That is an interesting comment from one of Thoreau's contemporaries, emphasizing the tension between the swamp and the city. We might all aim for "aboriginal civility"—being a nature person and yet cultivating our urbanity.

I take Alcott's use of the word *aboriginal*, which Emerson used as a key concept, to mean "deeply inborn" or "of one's essence." Its Latin roots mean "from the beginning" or "from one's origins." Perhaps it means "as basic as you can get." Thoreau had this sometimes charming and sometimes puzzling paradox in him: He certainly was a sylvan man, of the forest and the swamp, but he was also remarkably civil. He was comfortable with either a book or a hoe. Learn from this: Earnestly, be both earthy and intellectual.

48

THE BEASTS SPOKE

That Walt Whitman, of whom I wrote to you, is the most interesting fact to me at present. I have just read his edition (which he gave me) and it has done me more good than any reading for a long time. Perhaps I remember best the poem of Walt Whitman "An American and the Sun Down Poem"—There are 2 or 3 pieces in the book which are disagreeable, to say the least, simply sensual. He does not celebrate love at all—It is as if the beasts spoke . . . I found his poem exhilarating-encouraging . . . As for its sensuality . . . I do not so much wish that those parts were not written, as that men and women were so pure that they could read them without harm . . . I do not believe that all the sermons so called that have been preached in this land put together are equal to it for preaching.[1]

—Henry David Thoreau to Harrison
Gray Otis Blake, December 7, 1856

Walt Whitman renamed "The Sundown Poem," calling it "Crossing Brooklyn Ferry." It celebrates the people who crowd onto the ferries and cross into Brooklyn, a metaphor for all the people who cross into our lives and ferry out of them. He describes "the certainty of others, the life, love, sight, hearing of others." Thoreau was not so endeared of others, and certainly not charmed by a current of them rushing so thick and swift. Emerson observed, "Thoreau was not easy-going, it cost him nothing to say no and he often preferred solitude." The "other" he appreciated usually took animal form or grew near a tree and would not have been found on a ferry.

Thoreau's well-known, defining act was a solitary one: Leaving home, building a small cabin, establishing a lifestyle focused on animals, landscapes, bodies of water, and fish. He cherished being a self in solitude, relating more to nature than to people. His neighbors felt he was odd, although he did have many friends and participated in town life. He gave well-received talks at the local lyceum and surveyed land for many local farmers and business leaders. In Thoreau's time the population of Concord was two thousand, so it was not easy to be invisible anyway.

Setting out to write about Thoreau, I wondered if he was as sentimental a man as people make him out to be, living in his cabin and listening to the music of the trees. The first environmentalist. While reading him, I discovered that he was much more subtle and inventive. The other version, the Romantic in his canoe, would not be interested in Whitman, perhaps, but the Thoreau who writes about his daily experiences as a poet and in the special kind of prose he invented, would find a friend in *Leaves of Grass*. Whitman's powerful imagery rolls out like "the naked meat of the body," as he pictures it, or "the thin red jellies within you or within me." Thoreau's writing more philosophically evokes the red jellies of good ideas and fresh takes on the world in which we live. I think Thoreau's poetic prose would please Whitman.

Reading Whitman, he says, did Thoreau more good than "any reading for a long time." It is not so surprising that he would appreciate

Whitman, as Emerson did, not only for the grace of his language, but for the way he contemplates the human soul. Thoreau was engaged all his life at finding a view of human life that would give him a direction and a life work. He arrived at it by observing nature closely, while Whitman, living in Brooklyn, found it in the masses of people going about their lives, and especially in the ways they lived from their bodies inward to the soul. This was not Thoreau's way, unless you consider nature the world's body. It is clear anyway that Whitman's sensuality was not the selling point for Thoreau.

In this letter to his friend Blake, Thoreau tackles an issue at the heart of his appreciation for Whitman: his own sensual way of being in nature versus Whitman's turning to human sexuality for meaning. Thoreau lived sensually with the natural seasons, plant life, animals, birds, and even the human-made artifacts that were part of his landscape—the telegraph wires that made music and his cherished native arrowheads. Whitman's sensuality focused on the human body in an ecstatic way, as in these lines from his poem "I Sing the Body Electric":

> *Limitless limpid jets of love hot and enormous, quivering jelly of love, white-blow and delirious juice,*
> *Bridegroom night of love working surely and softly into the prostrate dawn,*
> *Undulating into the willing and yielding day,*
> *Lost in the cleave of the clasping and sweet-flesh'd day.*

Thoreau does not wish that such lines were not written, but that men and women could read them without harm. By harm, maybe he meant being disturbed by the images or entering an area—sexuality—that can be morally and emotionally challenging. He seems uncertain whether Whitman's highly sensuous writing has enough human meaning and is not just animal delight. Yet, in the end he supports Whitman and even claims, with strong sentiment, that not all the sermons that had been given so far in America could match the value of Whitman's writing.

Whitman took advantage of Emerson's enthusiastic support, publishing Emerson's initial words of endorsement, which were intended to be private. Emerson was not pleased, and his enthusiasm declined somewhat, although in the end he championed Whitman. He told Whitman that his concern was not moral as much as marketing. Would people accept Whitman's physical prose?

When you read Whitman's many long poems in which he moves firmly from physical delight to soul, you may understand how Whitman and Thoreau could understand each other. Whitman is heavy on the sensual, and Thoreau weighs in on sensuality in nature. Both were passionate, but in different ways. Both were expressing themselves in their full individuality, thus achieving the Emersonian ideal of self-reliance.

What does all of this say about our underlying issue in this book, learning from Thoreau's discovery of himself at Walden how to make a better world? Sensuality counts. It does not do to create a world where we study nature and harness it dispassionately for our egotistical purposes. It does not do to dissociate our sexuality from soul. What if we listen to the music of nature rather than translating nature into chemicals and products? What if we deepen our sexuality, affirming it strongly while tapping into it for a more enchanting and engaging way of life, moving like Whitman from sex to an ecstatic celebration of humanity?

I fully enjoy Whitman's sensual language. It thrills me. But for myself and my way of life, I prefer Thoreau's Artemisian, sylvan sensuality. I have much of his Artemis in me, the Greek goddess of reserve and purity. I don't want to offend Aphrodite in all her sexual sensuality, and I honor her in subtle ways, as I think Thoreau did.

He was sensual in the woods, on mountain trails, and on rivers. You can maintain your respect for both Artemis and Aphrodite by being sensual with some reserve or by expressing your sexuality in ways not so literal. Still, it is obvious that Thoreau preferred to visit the temple of Artemis.

In the letter sent to Blake, Thoreau is ambivalent about his feelings toward Whitman's overt sensuality. In the end he connects it to a new kind of spirituality that is in and of the world and inspired by a person's sexual nature. The idea is not to resolve the issue of purity and sensuality intellectually, but to embrace them both, with all their contradictions and paradoxes.

49

SOMEWHERE BETWEEN ME AND THEM

I think that the man of science makes this mistake, and the mass of mankind along with him: that you should cooly give your chief attention to the phenomenon which excites you as something independent on you, and not as it is related to you . . . It is the subject of the vision, the truth alone, that concerns me. The philosopher for whom rainbows, etc., can be explained away never saw them . . . the point of interest is somewhere between me and them.[1]

—Henry David Thoreau, journal entry, November 5, 1857

Thoreau was meticulous in his study of plant life, but he did not use scientific methods strictly. He leaned more toward eros than logos. Eros is the desire, connection, and magnetism that draws us into the world, logos our quest for understanding. Thoreau followed his natural inclinations and desires and expressed his observations in situ, as he came upon them in his personal activities. He developed relationships with the natural objects in his world and wrote about them as friends and neighbors. He said that you should get to know the natural world not in the abstract, but as the local world in which you live. He wanted an intimate relationship with the world, not a cool, remote understanding of it. Berry-picking, his alternative to scientific study, has an element of play in it, and that, too, is a sign of eros.

Science generally prides itself on its detachment, but Thoreau would not agree. Making a game of berry-picking is part of his method. When friends visit and kayak with us in our pond, they are clearly coming for pleasure, and in their pleasurable play they may learn about nature in a way not accessible to formal studies. We do not have to objectify the world to understand it. Thoreau's boating down a river was his method for earning about and befriending the natural world. Our intimacy with the natural world, our part in it and our love of it, all play roles in our attempts to know more about it.

I prefer the word *ecology* to *environmentalism*. *Ecology* has the Greek word *oikos* in the center of it, meaning "home." *Environmentalism*, a much longer and clumsier word, is from French and Latin words meaning "to turn around in." We might say "hanging around in." In ecology you find your home, one of the deepest experiences a human being can have. In environmentalism nature is where you can hang around.

The soft eroticism in Thoreau also showed itself in his way of befriending nature. He would go into it with music and the joy of boating and hiking and, whenever possible, berry-picking. He sought full experience of nature, and his way of being poetic, friendly, and playful was his method.

In this journal entry he says that it is a mistake to think that nature is independent from us and not related to us. We are born of the planet and therefore have true sibling relationships with other beings, including plant life. Our connection is family rather than resource. His success in training mice and chipmunks to come to him was not just the good outcome of a magic trick, but practicing natural science in his own engaged way and manifesting a serious yet playful friendship.

When Thoreau was out in nature, he felt a closeness and connection to the world around him. It is not a good idea, he says, to give a complete analysis of a rainbow without ever having seen one. That may be an exaggeration, and many scientists, if not most, love the natural world and that part of it that they study. But their method is not always playful and intimate. Thoreau offers us a challenge to do things differently and take the risk to include love and play in our serious studies.

NASA, too, could be more philosophical in a deep and engaging way, as they make expensive, challenging voyages into space and visiting other planets. I would like to see NASA consulting with natural theologians, since our penetration into the mysteries of the cosmos affects our image of the universe and therefore our conception of who we are. All of this goes back to Thoreau, who recommends a focus somewhere between the object of our study and us.

I am reminded of the German Romantic poet Novalis in a passage that could be applied to Thoreau's constant dictum that in nature we find ourselves: "The seat of the soul is there, where the inner world and the outer world touch. Where they permeate each other, the seat is in very point of the permeation."[2]

Today people consider mining minerals and other materials from planets and moons, another materialistic encroachment of space. This approach is like studying rainbows without looking at one. We don't know what we are doing, but we do it anyway. NASA could consult with artists and mystics, people who could bring a profound human sensitivity to the world we are just discovering and offer reasons for doing it. Or will we repeat what Christopher Columbus did in his explorations of the Caribbean—exploit new strange lands and bring loot home to the masters of economics, the king and queen, who crave material wealth?

For centuries people have allowed their lives to be guided by the movements of the planets and other celestial bodies and have even named them after gods and goddesses. The days of the week similarly have mythological names. All of this implies a mutual, intimate, and important connection between our private lives and celestial bodies.

"The point of interest is somewhere between me and them." When we investigate the world for its order and meaning, we could include both the natural world and our human situation. The object of our interest is in neither but is between them. We could bring some soul to science by constantly including our important human interests in our studies and by including philosophers, theologians, and artists in our scientific adventures. Emerson wrote: "Only the poet knows astronomy."

We get glimpses of in between science in astrology, alchemy, and cosmic music, which today are considered New Age, but were once legitimate forms of knowledge, if slightly to the side of the mainstream. To the poets and visual artists these "sciences" are finding legitimacy and are guiding us inward.

Many people in the throes of difficult emotions feel compelled to go to the sea, climb a mountain, or dig in the ground. Without thinking much about it, they go to nature with their troubles that seem to have no rational solution. Finding that spot between the world and the self, they are comforted, at least a little, and they may learn how to incorporate nature into their emotional lives.

It would help to reflect more seriously and specifically on all the things we do with our science and technology so that we might attend to the human element more fully, thus humanizing our science and in that way restoring our humanity. Eventually we may rediscover animism, the sense that nature is alive and even has personality. Our objectification of the natural world may be nothing more than a defensive maneuver against animism and against nature's power and subjectivity. It may also justify our exploitation of raw life in the natural realm.

The same development would also deepen the practice of medicine, which has surrendered to pure science. Naturally we have therapeutics in mind in medical research and practice, but we conceive medicine itself almost entirely as an objective science. We do not meet the body and the self at anywhere near a midpoint, where the two would be considered equal. Instead, we *apply* our science to the human, who becomes the subject of our investigations and applications.

In Greek mythology, Orpheus, one of the few to visit the Underworld in hopes to reason with death, played his stringed instrument and charmed the natural world. Thoreau went into nature and played his flute, an example for us how to live a more mythic life and also how to be in nature as a human being. He invites us to be Orphic in our approach to nature, doing our part to enchant the animals and plants, going fearlessly into the depth, the underworld, of all that we do.

50

A FINE EFFLUENCE

The mystery of the life of plants is kindred with that of our own lives, and the physiologist must not presume to explain their growth according to mechanical laws . . . The ultimate expression or fruit of any created thing is a fine effluence which only the most ingenuous worshipper perceives at a reverent distance from its surface even. . . . Only that intellect makes any progress toward conceiving of the essence which at the same time perceives the effluence.[1]

—Henry David Thoreau, journal entry, March 7, 1859

When I finished writing my comments on Thoreau's writings, I came across scholars saying that he became an empirical scientist in his later years, losing much of his transcendentalism. I was confused because in reading his journals, even in the last years—say, from the late 1850s until his death in 1862—I found the old transcendental Thoreau present. Then I found passages in David Robinson's penetrating book, *Natural Life: Thoreau's Worldly*

Transcendentalism, that resolved this issue with an emphasis on Thoreau's single word: *effluence.*

At the beginning of the selection we find the old theme: The lives of plants are kindred with our own lives. If we study nature, we should do it with ourselves along for the ride. Looking into the natural world is to look inside ourselves.

The word *effluence* means something "flowing from." Robinson relates this idea to Thoreau's interest in the aromas of nature, as when he suggests rubbing a handkerchief on an apple to get its fragrance. Thoreau went on his long, studious walks not only with his ears tuned to the music of the forest, but also with his famous prominent nose alert to the aromas flowing from the plants. The eyes are not central for the naturalist, as was made evident in Thoreau's enchanting walks in the moonlight.

Among the things flowing from plants in the forest and on the riverbanks are more abstract qualities that help a human being get along and find their way in life: beauty, efficiency, mutuality, and timing. Another word for effluence might be *emanation*. A spirit emanates from trees, plants, and even animals. Together these various kinds of spirit coalesce to make the spirit of the wilderness. You walk in a forest, take in the qualitative spirit of the vegetation and the creatures, and you are renewed and recreated. My Italian Renaissance source, Marsilio Ficino, recommends that, when you are depressed, walk by a body of water shimmering in the sunlight and absorb that special spirit.

If we want to learn from Thoreau how to solve our problems by deepening the human experience, we could approach the natural sciences through the effluences of nature and not only from its material components and processes. These are the intermediaries between the wilderness and the human sphere. The ancient Greeks would personify these effluences as gods and goddesses, daimons, and nymphs. I have found it easy to adopt the mythological names and look for Artemis in a forest or a naiad, a water nymph, by a pond. When Thoreau says that Walden Pond gave him an experience of Eden, he was also speaking mythologically.

When you walk in a forest or up a mountain, for example, you almost always notice the beauty around you. This implies that beauty is essential in a natural life, and if beauty is central in nature, it is central in human experience generally. In a forest, beauty is not accidental or unimportant. People walking in nature usually comment repeatedly on the beauty of the scene they are looking at. They may want to take photographs to bring that beauty home with them or set up an easel and make a painting. They want to capture the effluence.

Living in the woods and by water, I also learn about myself when I notice how the natural world is always changing. In mid-season—say, the middle of summer—you can enjoy a week or two of relative stability. Later, moving toward autumn, changes in the colors and weather will be dramatic. Plants, of course, as Thoreau noted in meticulous observations of local varieties, go through constant change, which can be compared to similar changes a year or more ago. This movement can help us humans notice the changes in ourselves as the year progresses. We are part of that sweep of change over time and in season.

We learn from trees to bend with the wind and to stand tall, and from flowers to show our beauty and survive in our delicacy. We discover in streams how to bend with resistance and, in Thoreau's witty observation, be deep in our shallowness. We learn from the weather to be tempestuous when necessary and balmy when possible. Butterflies teach us not to soar too high but to enjoy our low flights, and hawks and eagles demonstrate spreading our wings and going high.

These are generic lessons from nature, but if you were to go deep into the wilderness you would learn subtle lessons in living on this planet and being a person. That was Thoreau's destination when he opted for a cabin by a pond not far from his family home. He understood that gaining distance from the familiar and the structured does not have to be a literal escape but only a very small move in another direction.

This might be one of the great lessons to take from Walden Pond: A slight move from your standard life, especially into the primeval wild of nature, can reset your life and give it the elusive purpose you may have been looking for. Some people are shocked when they learn how close Walden Pond is to Concord. During his retreat Thoreau was not far from civilization or his family. But that is the idea. You can miniaturize your life, take a "long" trip just out of town and in that way give it a deeper, more poetic meaning.

It is not enough to be purposeless in your excursions. You can sense the effluences of oaks and ferns and chipmunks. You open your inner eyes to the invisibles in the world around you, including the special spirits that emanate from every aspect of nature. They are food for your soul. You look for effluences that are special to you and sometimes unique. One of the world's natural wonders that serves as a healing effluence to me is the Cliffs of Moher in Ireland. With my wife and children, I used to spend time in County Clare, with its narrow stone-lined roads and ancient antiquities. They would sit at the edge of a cliff and sketch or paint while I, with my anxiety about heights, would worry for their safety. But my heart, or whichever organ is involved, was filled with wonder and a huge sense of sheer being.

As we travel, we are gathering the effluences of much loved or unknown places, enriching our interior lives. That is one way to understand Thoreau's often quoted line: I have traveled in Concord. He lived in and near Concord, but without leaving it, he traveled the world. Emily Dickinson, so much like Thoreau in her garden and among the

Amherst hills, knew this secret of geographical exploration and time travel.

> I never saw a Moor—
> I never saw the Sea—
> Yet know I how the Heather looks
> And what a Billow be.[2]

The effluence of nature includes the emotions, memories, and fantasies it stirs in us. In this sense, one of the main reasons to go into the natural world is to receive its fine perfume, its misting of spirit.

Thoreau challenges us to go into nature, of whatever kind, and receive the mysterious truths that pour out of it and enrich the humans who touch the plants and sit in the cooling shadow of a tree's crown. Do not merely study nature—be in it and accept its gifts, in whatever form you may find them. Be open to new possibilities and quiet, hardly visible truths. Allow yourself to be transformed by nature, as it is given to you. Use your imagination and do not demand that everything be actual and literal. Nature will overshadow you in all its faint forms. It helps if you do not only look but embrace and internalize what nature is about. As some have said, Thoreau was always on a vision quest, and that could be our purpose as we walk eyes open through the green density of a pristine forest.

ACKNOWLEDGMENTS

In my home we often say that it feels like a creative arts center. My wife, Joan Hanley, paints expertly. My daughter, Siobhán or Ajeet, is a remarkable musician, painter, and writer. My stepson, Abe, is a genius architect and designer. I never stop writing, except to play the piano and wash dishes. My debt to these three remarkable people in relation to this book, and of course to life in general, is beyond saying. What fires us is the love among us.

Our neighbors and friends are also incredibly creative. Andrew Krivak lives next door, and he is destined to be a great American novelist. Our conversations keep me excited about books. His wife, Amelia Dunlop, is another gifted neighbor who works a special magic on my creative life. Another brilliant couple, Patrice and Gary Pinette, generously befriended us when we landed in New Hampshire thirty years ago and have inspired us ever since with their talent in poetry and music. Gary and I share an intense interest in psychotherapy and often like to talk about it somewhat irreverently but seriously. Patrice is a born poet with an exquisite appreciation for language and imagery. We have spent many hours discussing poems, poets, and language. She has a special interest in Thoreau and other transcendentalists, and so her responses to my writing have been especially penetrating.

I have not met many of the devoted scholars of Thoreau. I have exchanged messages with Jeffrey Cramer, whose name you see often in this book. His annotated edition of *Walden* and selections from Thoreau's journals, *I to Myself*, are beautiful, useful, and altogether extraordinary volumes. I love to hold these and other books of his in my hands and use them for my own writing. I am also overwhelmed with the insights and style of David Robinson's *Natural Life*. As I prepared to write I was stunned by the quality of books on Thoreau that I found, including the biographies. I'll just mention the work of Laura Dassow Walls, Kevin Dann, and Walter Harding. I hesitate to make this list because I will certainly overlook excellent writings. The list is vast.

I owe some insights to conversations with Craig Stockwell, an incredibly inventive painter and golf partner, and with Humberto Ramirez, another splendid painter and conversationalist. The support of Bob Callahan and Jill Goldman-Callahan, old friends and Concord residents, kept me going at faint moments. Lucy Thomas has long encouraged me in all my writing, but especially for this book.

As I write this remembrance I am in my mid-eighties, and I want to say how much it has meant to me to have the personal and professional support of my agent Todd Shuster, who has advised me at this moment in my career with warmth and understanding. Thanks, too, to his team of Jack Haug and Anna Shumway. I still value the friendship and advice of Hugh Van Dusen and Bill Shinker, continuing from the old days.

I'm happy now to be in the brilliant hands of Jessica Case and Claiborne Hancock at Pegasus Books. I am grateful for their trust and hope in my work.

Notes

Epigraph

1 Horace Traubel, *With Walt Whitman in Camden*, 1914

1: Blue Angels

1 Jeffrey S. Cramer, ed., *Walden: A Fully Annotated Edition* (Yale University Press, 2004), 112.

2: Fluttering

1 Jeffrey S. Cramer, ed., *I to Myself: An Annotated Selection from the Journal of Henry David Thoreau* (Yale University Press, 2007), 30.

2 Helen Vendler, *Dickinson: Selected Poems and Commentaries* (Harvard University Press, 2010), 27.

3: Etherealized by a Mountain

1 Jeffrey S. Cramer, ed., *I to Myself: An Annotated Selection from the Journal of Henry David Thoreau* (Yale University Press, 2007), 99.

4: Inorganic and Lumpish

1 Bradford Torrey, ed., *The Journal of Henry David Thoreau*, vol. 9 (Peregrine Smith Books, 1984), 246.

2 Jeffrey S. Cramer, ed., *Walden: A Fully Annotated Edition* (Yale University Press, 2004), 88.

3 Torrey, *The Journal of Henry David Thoreau*, January 16, 1860.

5: The Sound of the Rooster

1 Jeffrey S. Cramer, ed., *Essays by Henry D. Thoreau: A Fully Annotated Edition* (Yale University Press, 2013), 278.

6: The Sacred Swamp

1 Jeffrey S. Cramer, ed., *Essays by Henry D. Thoreau: A Fully Annotated Edition* (Yale University Press, 2013), 262.

7: A Dose of Myself

1 Jeffrey S. Cramer, ed., *Essays by Henry D. Thoreau: A Fully Annotated Edition* (Yale University Press, 2013), 347.

8: Accidents

1 Bradford Torrey, ed., *The Journal of Henry David Thoreau*, vol. 12 (Peregrine Smith Books, 1984), 39.

9: Consult Your Genius

1 Robert N. Hudspeth, ed., *The Correspondence of Henry D. Thoreau, Volume 2: 1849–1856* (Princeton University Press, 2018), 122–23.

10: Dipped Toast

1 Bradford Torrey, ed., *The Journal of Henry David Thoreau*, vol. 9 (Peregrine Smith Books, 1984), 283–84.

11: The Civilized Apple Tree

1 Jeffrey S. Cramer, ed., *Essays by Henry D. Thoreau: A Fully Annotated Edition* (Yale University Press, 2013), 319.

2 Bradford Torrey, ed., *The Journal of Henry David Thoreau*, vol. 9 (Peregrine Smith Books, 1984), 146.

12: A Broad Margin to My Life

1 Jeffrey S. Cramer, ed., *Walden: A Fully Annotated Edition* (Yale University Press, 2004), 108.

2 Cramer, *Walden: A Fully Annotated Edition*, 108n5.

3 Shunryu Suzuki, *Zen Mind, Beginner's Mind* (Weatherhill, 1973), 49.

13: The Sacred Art of Farming

1 Jeffrey S. Cramer, ed., *Walden: A Fully Annotated Edition* (Yale University Press, 2004), 160.

2 Wendell Berry, "Economy and Pleasure," in *Sex, Economy, Freedom & Community* (Counterpoint Press, 1993).

3 Wallace Stevens, *The Collected Poems of Wallace Stevens* (Alfred A. Knopf, 1971), 473.

14: Walden in Eden

1 Jeffrey S. Cramer, ed., *Walden: A Fully Annotated Edition* (Yale University Press, 2004), 174.

2 David Mikics, *The Annotated Emerson* (Harvard University Press, 2012), 31.

3 Jeffrey S. Cramer, ed., *Walden: A Fully Annotated Edition* (Yale University Press, 2004), 180.

15: Be Cold and Hungry

1 Bradford Torrey, ed., *The Journal of Henry David Thoreau*, vol. 9 (Peregrine Smith Books, 1984), 198.

2 Ralph Waldo Emerson, "Thoreau," *The Atlantic*, August, 1862.

16: The Cold Blood of the Gods

1 Robert N. Hudspeth, ed., *The Correspondence of Henry D. Thoreau, Volume 2: 1849–1856*, (Princeton University Press, 2018), 388.

2 Jeffrey S. Cramer, ed., *I to Myself: An Annotated Selection from the Journal of Henry David Thoreau* (Yale University Press, 2007), 39.
3 David V. Erdman, ed., *The Complete Poetry and Prose of William Blake* (University of California Press, 1982), 39.

17: Clodhopper that I Am
1 Robert N. Hudspeth, ed., *The Correspondence of Henry D. Thoreau, Volume 2: 1849–1856*, (Princeton University Press, 2018), 404, 434–35.
2 Wendell Berry, *The Hidden Wound* (Counterpoint, 2010), 101.

18: The Fern Scriptures
1 Jeffrey S. Cramer, ed., *I to Myself: An Annotated Selection from the Journal of Henry David Thoreau* (Yale University Press, 2007), 405.

19: The Apple Tree Building
1 Jeffrey S. Cramer, ed., *Walden: A Fully Annotated Edition* (Yale University Press, 2004), 189.
2 Richard Higgins, "Thoreau's Places," *Thoreau Society Bulletin*, no. 314 (Summer 2021), 5.
3 Joel Myerson, *Cambridge Companion to Henry David Thoreau* (Cambridge University Press, 1995), 211, n. 9.

20: The Eyelids of the Day
1 Robert N. Hudspeth, ed., *The Correspondence of Henry D. Thoreau, Volume 2: 1849–1856*, (Princeton University Press, 2018), 122.

21: The Hoary Bloom
Jeffrey S. Cramer, ed., *I to Myself: An Annotated Selection from the Journal of Henry David Thoreau* (Yale University Press, 2007), 277.
1 Bradford Torrey, ed., *The Journal of Henry David Thoreau*, vol. 10 (Peregrine Smith Books, 1984), 160–61.
2 James Hillman, *The Force of Character* (Random House, 1999), 199.
3 Cramer, *I to Myself*, 277.

22: The Heavens Withdraw
1 Bradford Torrey, ed., *The Journal of Henry David Thoreau*, vol. 9 (Peregrine Smith Books, 1984), 283–84.

23: I Am Stone
1 Bradford Torrey, ed., *The Journal of Henry David Thoreau*, vol. 3 (Peregrine Smith Books, 1984), 147.
2 Paul Ward, "How Humans Deal With and Survive Extreme Cold," Cool Antarctica, https://www.coolantarctica.com/Antarctica%20fact%20file/science/cold_humans.php.

24: Lapse of Time
1 Bradford Torrey, ed., *The Journal of Henry David Thoreau*, vol. 9 (Peregrine Smith Books, 1984), 311.

25: Imported Woods
1 Jeffrey S. Cramer, ed., *Essays by Henry D. Thoreau: A Fully Annotated Edition* (Yale University Press, 2013), 248, 244.

2 Lawwrence Rosenwald, ed., *Emerson: Selected Journals, 1841-1877* (Library of America, 2010), 129.

26: The Brows of the Earth

1 Jeffrey S. Cramer, ed., *I to Myself: An Annotated Selection from the Journal of Henry David Thoreau* (Yale University Press, 2007), 99, 430.

27: The Music of the World

1 Laura Dassow Walls, *Henry David Thoreau: A Life* (University of Chicago Press, 2017), 267.
2 Bradford Torrey, ed., *The Journal of Henry David Thoreau*, vol. 9 (Peregrine Smith Books, 1984), 222.
3 Jeffrey S. Cramer, ed., *Walden: A Fully Annotated Edition* (Yale University Press, 2004), 154.
4 Jeffrey S. Cramer, ed., *I to Myself: An Annotated Selection from the Journal of Henry David Thoreau* (Yale University Press, 2007), 492.
5 Cramer, *Walden: A Fully Annotated Edition*, 114.
6 Cramer, *Walden: A Fully Annotated Edition*, 115.
7 Cramer, *I to Myself*, 28.
8 Homeric Hymn to Pan, trans. Thomas Moore. Unpublished.

28: Dried Fungus

1 Robert N. Hudspeth, ed., *The Correspondence of Henry D. Thoreau, Volume 2: 1849–1856*, (Princeton University Press, 2018), 470.

29: Organic Earth

1 Bradford Torrey, ed., *The Journal of Henry David Thoreau*, vol. 3 (Peregrine Smith Books, 1984), 165–66.
2 Torrey, *The Journal of Henry David Thoreau.*
3 Plotinus, *Enneads*, trans. Stephen MacKenna (Penguin Books, 1991).
4 Plotinus, *Enneads*, 318.

30: Filibustering Toward Heaven

Bradley P. Dean, ed., *Henry David Thoreau: Letters to a Spiritual Seeker* (W. W. Norton, 2004), 53.
1 Dean, *Henry David Thoreau: Letters to a Spiritual Seeker*, 82–83.

31: A Respectable Distance

1 Jeffrey S. Cramer, ed., *I to Myself: An Annotated Selection from the Journal of Henry David Thoreau* (Yale University Press, 2007), 60.
2 David Mikics, *The Annotated Ralph Waldo Emerson* (Harvard University Press, 2012), 105.
3 Mikics, *The Annotated Ralph Waldo Emerson*, 105.
4 Bradley P. Dean, *Letters to a Spiritual Seeker* (New York: W. W. Norton, 2004), 50.

32: Our Cousins the Cats

1 Bradford Torrey, ed., *The Journal of Henry David Thoreau*, vol. 9 (Peregrine Smith Books, 1984), 178.
2 Jeffrey S. Cramer, ed., *I to Myself: An Annotated Selection from the Journal of Henry David Thoreau* (Yale University Press, 2007), 101.
3 Cramer, *I to Myself*, 199.

33: Every Town Needs a Park

1 Jeffrey S. Cramer, ed., *I to Myself: An Annotated Selection from the Journal of Henry David Thoreau* (Yale University Press, 2007), 405.
2 Mircea Eliade, *Myth, Dreams, and Mysteries*, trans. Philip Mairet (New York: Harper & Row, 1957), 31.
3 Eliade, *Myths, Dreams, and Mysteries*, 31.

34: My Own Sacraments

1 Jeffrey S. Cramer, ed., *I to Myself: An Annotated Selection from the Journal of Henry David Thoreau* (Yale University Press, 2007), 40–41.
2 Euripides, *Bakkhai*, trans. Anne Carson (New Directions, 2017), 12–13.

35: My Inner Eastward Mountains

1 Bradley P. Dean, ed., *Henry David Thoreau: Letters to a Spiritual Seeker* (W. W. Norton, 2004), 159.
2 Jeffrey S. Cramer, ed., *I to Myself: An Annotated Selection from the Journal of Henry David Thoreau* (Yale University Press, 2007), 410.
3 Cramer, *I to Myself*, 28.
4 Cramer, *I to Myself*, 109.

36: The Philosophy of Wood

1 Jeffrey S. Cramer, ed., *Walden: A Fully Annotated Edition* (Yale University Press, 2004), 415–16.

37: The Mouth of a Reptile

1 Bradford Torrey, ed., *The Journal of Henry David Thoreau*, vol. 2 (Peregrine Smith Books, 1984), 444.
2 Jeffrey S. Cramer, ed., *I to Myself: An Annotated Selection from the Journal of Henry David Thoreau* (Yale University Press, 2007), 277.
3 Bradley P. Dean, ed., *Henry David Thoreau: Letters to a Spiritual Seeker* (W. W. Norton, 2004), 142.

38: The Poetry of Fish

1 Jeffrey S. Cramer, ed., *I to Myself: An Annotated Selection from the Journal of Henry David Thoreau* (Yale University Press, 2007), 374–76.
2 Edward O. Wilson, *Biophilia* (Harvard University Press, 1984), 28–29.
3 C. G. Jung, *Mysterium Coniunctionis*, trans. R.F.C. Hull (Princeton: Princeton University Press, 1970), 51.

39: Room for Thought

1 Jeffrey S. Cramer, ed., *Walden: A Fully Annotated Edition* (Yale University Press, 2004), 136.

40: Not Spiritual, but Natural

1 Henry David Thoreau, *A Week on the Concord and Merrimack Rivers*, ed. Carl Hovde, et al. (Princeton: Princeton University Press, 1980), 379.

41: A Rich and Fertile Mystery

Bradford Torrey, ed., *The Journal of Henry David Thoreau*, vol. 2 (Peregrine Smith Books, 1984), 270. Jeffrey S. Cramer, ed., *I to Myself: An Annotated Selection from the Journal of Henry David Thoreau* (Yale University Press, 2007), 68.

1 Carl Bode, ed., *The Portable Emerson* (Penguin Books, 1981), 87.
2 Bode, *The Portable Emerson*, 87.
3 Robert Gittings, ed., *Letters of John Keats* (Oxford University Press, 1970), 249.

42: Soul Sculpting

1 Jeffrey S. Cramer, ed., *Walden: A Fully Annotated Edition* (Yale University Press, 2004), 213.
2 Plotinus, *Enneads*, trans. Stephen MacKenna (Penguin Books, 1991), 54.
3 Robert Gittings, *Letters of John Keats* (Oxford University Press, 1970), 36–37.
4 Friedrich Nietzsche, *The Gay Science* (Ernst Schmeitzner, 1882).

43: Slight Impulses

1 Jeffrey S. Cramer, ed., *I to Myself: An Annotated Selection from the Journal of Henry David Thoreau* (Yale University Press, 2007), 276–77.

44: On Tiptoe

1 Jeffrey S. Cramer, ed., *Walden: A Fully Annotated Edition* (Yale University Press, 2004), 102.

45: A Village A University

1 Jeffrey S. Cramer, ed., *Walden: A Fully Annotated Edition* (Yale University Press, 2004), 106–7.

46: The Walden Pond Society

1 Bradford Torrey, ed., *The Journal of Henry David Thoreau*, vol. 9 (Peregrine Smith Books, 1984), 331.

47: What Makes Me Rich

1 Bradford Torrey, ed., *The Journal of Henry David Thoreau*, vol. 9 (Peregrine Smith Books, 1984), 350.
2 Torrey, *The Journal of Henry David Thoreau*, vol. 2, 228.

48: The Beasts Spoke

1 Robert N. Hudspeth, ed., *The Correspondence of Henry D. Thoreau, Volume 2: 1849–1856*, (Princeton University Press, 2018), 488–89.

49: Somewhere Between Me and Them

1 Bradford Torrey, ed., *The Journal of Henry David Thoreau*, vol. 10 (Peregrine Smith Books, 1984), 164–65.
2 Arthur Versluis, transl., *Novalis: Pollen and Fragments* (Phanes Press, 1989), 15.

50: A Fine Effluence

1 Jeffrey S. Cramer, ed., *I to Myself: An Annotated Selection from the Journal of Henry David Thoreau* (Yale University Press, 2007), 386.
2 Thomas H. Johnson, ed., *The Complete Poems of Emily Dickinson* (Little Brown, 1960), 480.